CONTENTS

PAGE

2 .... DISCLAIMER

3 .... PART 1 - ABOUT THE AUTHOR

4-6 .... PART 2 - INTRODUCTION

7-10 .... PART 3 - The Home Health Care Nurse

11-13 .... PART 4 - Trends In Home Health Care

14-55 .... PART 5 - Special Procedures and quipment

56-63 .... PART 6 - Safety in the Home

64-65 .... Disaster Planning In Home Care

66-68 .... Bibliography

69-88 .... Appendix

89-94 .... Notes

On-the-go Vitals™ presents Book: "The Nurse's Guide to Home Health Care"
©All Rights Reserved
http://www.allhealthacademy.com

DISCLAIMER

On-the-go Vitals™ presents…

THE NURSE'S GUIDE TO HOME HEALTH CARE

©All Rights Reserved.

No part of this book may be reproduced without the written consent of the writer/publisher.
September 19, 2012.

You have purchased this book for personal use. You cannot distribute this book to anyone or any entity. This book does not include any resale rights whatsoever or private label licensing.

This book was written and produced by Averel Carby, RN, owner operator of Averel Carby Home Health Care, LLC and allhealthacademy.com.

The content herein is meant to be a general overview of home health care, and home health care procedures. It is not intended to be any detailed guidelines or standards. Please follow Doctors' orders, State, and Agency policies and procedures.

PART I

ABOUT THE AUTHOR

I am Averel Carby, registered nurse and founder of All Health Academy. My hospital experiences include acute Rehabilitation, recovery room (PACU), and oncology. The other areas of my nursing career are nurse care coordinator, and home health care nursing, the latter for fifteen years.

As a home health care nurse I have worked at the besides of countless individuals, and their families, providing one-on-one care. I am currently an Agency for Persons with Disabilities (APD) provider, offering education and coaching to group home providers.

You may contact me at the address and phone number below. I look forward to hearing from you:

All Health Academy
Averel Carby Home Health Care, LLC
561-574-4348
PO Box 211122
Royal Palm Beach, FL 33421

PART 2

INTRODUCTION

My reason for writing this nursing handbook is to attempt to address the need for education and support to the home health care nurse.

It was only fifteen years ago I first graduated from nursing school. There was little focus on home health care nursing in the curriculum. Consequently, when I decided to make this area of nursing a career, I had limited resources to turn to for the training and support I needed. I did receive some orientation from the agency I first worked for, but I felt that it was just not enough to dispel the apprehension I had.

With the pace of traditional hospital nursing being so fast, we sometimes find ourselves wondering if we are really able to make that strong nurse-patient connection.

At the beginning of your nursing education, you probably had a different expectation of the amount of time you would spend at the bedside with your patients.

As time went on and you gained more clinical experience, your expectation began to shift. But the true shift occurred when you hit the floor as a new nurse.

In most nursing specialties the patient-nurse ratio makes it difficult to connect on the level you would like to with your patients. There is just not enough time in the shift, with the amount of work you have to do. You often feel like you are rushing in and out of patients rooms in a hurry to "get it all done". This can leave you with the desire to connect more with patients.

This is precisely one of the reasons I started doing home care nursing. I realized it was an opportunity to spend more time with each patient. The setting is usually more relaxed and so there is a greater chance of connecting with the patient and family members. Not having much time at the bedside with patients while working in facilities was not a good situation for me.

Being in the home has the added benefit of being in the client's environment. Sometimes this can also be a disadvantage if the home setting is challenging, but many times it is not the case. I cherish the times I have been able to really bond with my patients and their families in their most comfortable environment.

Transitioning from facility nurse, to home care nurse was a great decision for me, since it suited my personality and working preference. The transition was not one hundred percent smooth. The home is obviously different, and I had no guidance like the information in this handbook offers. Nevertheless, if I had to do it all over again, I would. It is a decision I am glad I made.

Do you think maybe it is time for you to explore your options in home health care nursing?

PART 3

THE HOME HEALTH CARE NURSE

Home health care, or health care, are terms used to refer to any kind of care service provided in a patient's home by non-skilled person, or a health care professional. There is a growing movement to distinguish between home health care, meaning skilled nursing care, and Home Care, meaning non-skilled care (Wikipedia 2012).

The home health care nurse may be a LPN (Licensed Practical Nurse), or RN (Registered Nurse). Home care makes it possible for patients to remain in their own home rather than in a nursing home or other institution. The services provided in the home may be a combination of professional health care services such as physical therapy, medical or psychological assessment, occupational therapy, or speech therapy. Wound care, disease management and education, and medication teaching may also be provided as applicable.

The number of children with life-threatening, life-limiting and chronic conditions has increased drastically within the past decade (K.Cervisio 2010). Consequently, the need for home health care nurses has greatly increased.

This area of nursing is rewarding, and is an important part of the health care industry. Many of the clients who have chronic conditions and are at home need to have skilled caregivers due to the complexities involved in their day-to-day care. For example, many depend on ventilators for life support; they are considered vent dependent.

Some are receiving intravenous therapy, or may have other medical issues that require the constant assessment and intervention of a licensed professional.

Home health care nurses provide a wide range of services to clients and their families. These services include assessing the home environment, caring about the families, and constantly teaching them about their family members' diseases and certain interventions which they are able to provide for their loved ones.

These nurses also may need to address psychosocial issues of the family unit, and refer them to appropriate services in the community. Home health care nurses must be able to work independently. They may supervise home health aides.

Maybe you are reading this and would like to know how you may become a home health care nurse. Well, you will need to complete an Associate degree, or bachelor's degree program in nursing. These programs will provide in-class and clinical experience that will enable you to become an RN (Registered Nurse). An LPN can also be a home health care nurse. The study for LPN (Licensed Practical Nurse) may be obtained at a vocational school. The LPN program takes approximately 13 months to complete, and provides the student with nursing knowledge to qualify for employment as a nurse in the home.

Obtaining employment in home health is usually through home health agencies. They may be found online by doing a search.

Ask nurses who you know have worked through an agency to help you choose which one would suite your needs. You should seek agencies that care about their employees as well as their clients. Nurses who have worked with agencies will be able to help you make an informed decision about choosing an agency.

Make sure you ask a lot of questions at your orientation. The supervisor is usually willing to provide the training needed to enable you to be prepared before you actually begin working. You will also be doing yourself a favor by obtaining a good orientation. Take notes at the orientation (there is a section just for notes at the back of this manual).

PART 4

TRENDS IN HOME HEALTH CARE

Employment in home health care nursing is expected to grow rapidly. This is due, unfortunately, to the growing number of persons with disabilities, preference for care in the home, and technological advances to make it possible to bring complex treatments into the home (Mayo Clinic 2012). The career outlook for the next decade is strong, due largely to the aging Boomer generation who will need more health care as they become older (Online Education Database 2012). Recent legislation reforming healthcare also gives the home health care sector the opportunity to obtain a larger share of the health care industry (Wyatt Matas & Associates 2010).

The National Association for Home Care & Hospice (NAHC) produced a legislative agenda called "The 2013 Legislative Blueprint for Action". This document contains a discussion of NAHC's priorities and other important issues and recommendations relating to home care and hospice.

It was prepared through a series of meetings with home care and hospice professionals, State association members, and a survey of the NAHC members. The agenda has been reviewed by the Government Affairs Committee and was approved by the NAHC Board of Directors at its 2012 meeting.

NAHC believes that quality home care and hospice are the right of every American. NAHC also believes that home care and hospice are humane and cost-effective alternatives to institutionalization. "Home care and hospice reinforce and supplement the care provided by family members and friends and encourage maximum independence of thought and functioning, as well as preservation of human dignity" (National Association for Home Care & Hospice 2012). It is the hope of NAHC that this document will be helpful to the Congress in its deliberations, resulting in the enactment of legislation to improve the quality of life for Americans needing home health care and Hospice.

According to Wyatt Matas & Associates, an investment banking firm, home health care thrives with healthcare reform.

That is the title of a paper written in 2010 as follow-up to another paper titled "The Delineation of Healthcare: The Natural Evolution of a Healthy Industry". Wyatt Matas & Associates wrote that as a result of the overhaul of healthcare signed into law in 2010 by President Obama, a new Medicare reimbursement penalty for hospitals with high avoidable readmission rates and economic incentives created by the Independence at Home Act (IAH) will force the home care sector to embrace the larger healthcare sector in order to thrive. This new legislative framework places home care in position to be the solution to the problems plaguing the entire healthcare industry. Home care agencies will now have a unique opportunity to provide value to the health care system while at the same time earning significant financial gains (Wyatt Matas & Associates 2010).

PART 5

SPECIAL PROCEDURES AND EQUIPMENT

When you receive an assignment to work in the home, the agency should provide orientation. This may include mandatory CEU's, and CPR certification required by the Board of Nursing in your State. There may also be in-services on the operation and care of equipment, and the care of clients with certain procedures on the body. These could be tracheostomies, apnea monitors, ventilators, or gastrostomy tubes and feeding pumps, to name a few. The following are the care of some procedures and equipment of clients in the home.

The Tracheostomy Tube

People of any age may need to have a tracheostomy. A client may require a tracheostomy tube for several reasons, which may include the following:

- Congenital defect of the upper airway

- Removal of the larynx because of cancer

- Spinal cord injuries

- Neuromuscular diseases causing paralysis, or weakening of the muscles and nerves involved in breathing.

The client who is home from the hospital with a new tracheostomy will have orders from a physician for its care. There will also be follow-up appointments with the surgeon, and usually the first few tracheostomy changes will be done by the physician or surgeon.

The care of the client with a tracheostomy tube requires special skills by the home care nurse. He or she will need to know about the parts of the tracheostomy, its placement or position, care of the tube, and the care of the tracheostomy site.

The Outer Cannula of the Tracheostomy

The outer cannula is the main part of the tracheostomy tube. It is maintained in place by the trach tie or holder which goes around the client's neck.

Some trach tubes have an inflatable cuff around the end of the tube. The cuff makes a seal around the tracheal wall when it is inflated (see Figures 1 - 3 below). This helps to prevent aspiration of oral secretions in the airway, and prevents escape of air through the mouth.

Patients on ventilators, pediatric patients, and those who do not have problems swallowing usually do not require a cuff.

Inner Cannula

The inner cannula fits into the outer cannula and is locked in place. Some trach tubes have inner cannulas. To prevent mucus build up and plugging, the inner cannula must be removed and cleaned.

Obturator

The obturator helps to make insertion of the trach tube smoother. It has a tip that is rounded, and sticks out of the end of the outer cannula, which prevents any trauma from occurring as the trach tube is inserted. **THE OBTURATOR MUST BE REMOVED AS SOON AS THE TRACH TUBE IS INSERTED. THE AIRWAY IS OCCLUDED WHILE IT IS IN PLACE, AND THE CLIENT CANNOT BREATHE.**

Deflate And Inflate The Cuff

Withdraw a little air until there is a slight leak at the end of inspiration. This minimal leak technique is used to limit the amount of air that is placed in the cuff against the tracheal wall.

The inflated cuff makes a seal to the airway so the patient may get the prescribed amount of air ordered by the Doctor. The pressure must be monitored to prevent any damage to the tracheal wall.

The minimal occluding volume is another technique which may be used to check the cuff pressure. This is done by putting enough air into the cuff so no leak is heard during inspiration. When using a manometer, a cuff pressure reading of 25 cm H_2O is preferred (Breath of Life 2009).

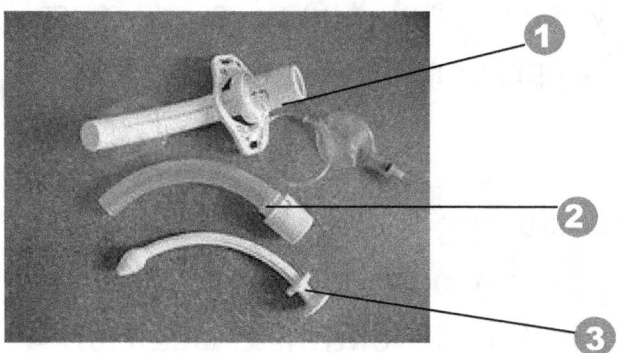

Figure 1– Cuffed Tracheostomy tube

1 – Outer cannula (notice that there is a fine tube attached to a balloon, for inflating and deflating the cuff at the end of the tube, using a small syringe that fits on the top of the balloon)

2 – Inner cannula

3 - Obturator

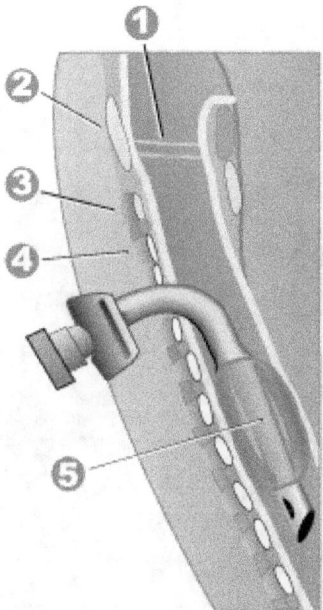

Figure 2 - Cuffed Tracheostomy tube

1 - Vocal folds

2 - Thyroid cartilage

3 - Cricoid cartilage

4 - Tracheal rings

5 - Balloon cuff (inflated)

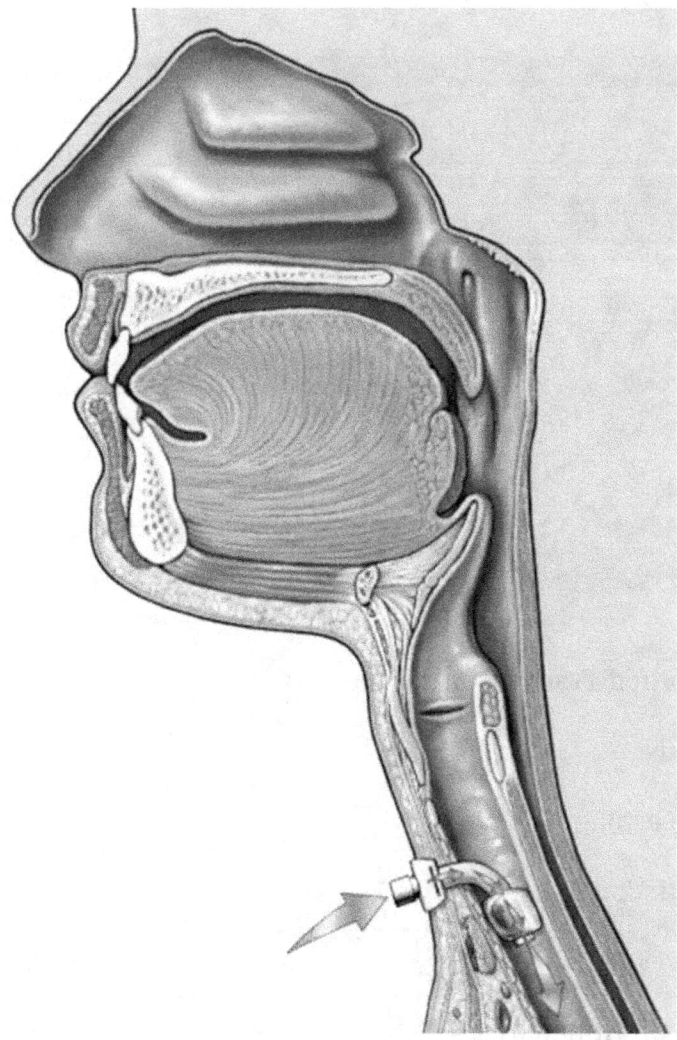

Figure 3– CUFFED TRACH

The pediatric, cuffed, Bivona tracheostomy tube is shown in Figure 4 below. The obturator is inserted into the cannula from the top. There is no inner cannula. The flange is across the top, and the slits are seen on both ends to hold the trach tie in place around the client's neck. At the end of the cannula is the deflated cuff. To the left is a fine tube and balloon, with connection to place a syringe for inflating and deflating the cuff. This type of trach is usually changed monthly, or as needed due to obstructive mucus.

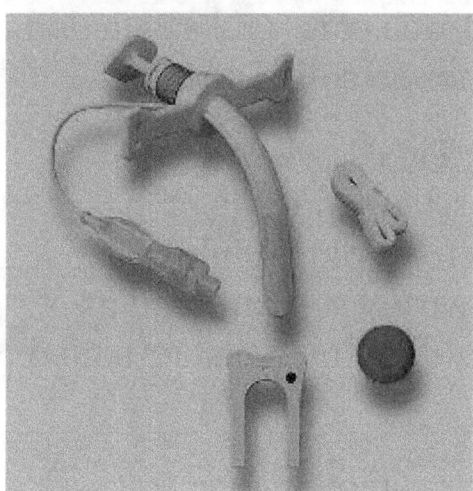

Figure 4 - Cuffed Bivona Tracheostomy Tube (Pediatric)

Tracheostomy Care

Keep the stoma and the trach tube clean. This should be done at least two times per day and as needed. The inner cannula, around the trach tube, and stoma should be cleaned. Clean technique is used. Change the trach tube each month, using sterile technique.

It is important to wash hands using good hand-washing technique, to prevent infection. Always wear gloves when handling trach tubes.

Tracheostomy Dressing

A dressing is placed around the trach tube to protect the patient's skin, and should be changed when doing trach care, and as needed. The dressing should not be soiled or moist.

Tracheostomy Tube Ties

The ties are used to prevent shifting or movement of the trach, keeping it in place. Change the ties daily with trach care and as needed. The ties should not be moist or soiled.

Changing The Trach Tie

- You need suction equipment, and trach tie.

- Wash your hands.

- While holding the trach in place, take the old tie off. Insert the end of the new tie into the hole of the outer flange of the trach tube.

- Place the other end into the slit of the other side of the trach flange.

- Tightly secure the tie to hold the trach tube in place securely. You should be able to place two fingers under the tie holder to make sure it is not too tight. Wash your hands.

How To Clean The Inner Cannula
- Keep the trach tube inner cannula clean and without dried secretions to prevent occlusion of the trach tube, and prevent the patient from breathing properly.

- Turn the inner cannula to the left or counter-clockwise in order to remove it.

- You may need to pinch the clip on the top of the inner cannula if it has a clip in order to remove it.

- Change the inner cannula daily. If you are using a non-disposable one, use sterile technique to clean it.

Tracheostomy Inner Cannula Change/Site Care
Use sterile technique to minimize infections (Breath of Life 2009). The following equipment will be in the sterile tracheostomy cleaning kit:

- Sterile tray
- Sterile field
- Sterile brush
- Sterile 4x4 gauze pads
- Sterile pipe cleaners
- Sterile gloves
- Sterile dressing pads
- Sterile trach ties

Have on hand:
- Clean inner cannula
- Hydrogen Peroxide
- Sterile water
- Sterile suction catheter
- Suction machine
- Ambu bag

Procedure:
- Wash your hands

- Open the sterile kit and provide a sterile field on work area.

- Pour the hydrogen peroxide in one tray, and the sterile water in the other side.

- Place the sterile glove on your dominant hand.

- Remove the items from the kit with the sterile gloved hand, and put them on the sterile field. Suction the patient.

- Disconnect the patient from the vent with your non-sterile hand.

- Unlock and remove the inner cannula with your non-sterile hand, and place it in the tray with the hydrogen peroxide to soak, If using a non-disposable inner cannula.

- Insert a clean inner cannula into the trach tube and reconnect the patient to the vent.

- Use the sterile brush to clean the inner Cannula.

- Rinse the inner cannula with the sterile water.

- Use the sterile 4x4 to dry the inner cannula.

- Store the clean inner cannula in a covered Container.

- Suction the patient as needed.

- Remove the soiled trach dressing using the non-sterile hand.

- Clean the skin with a gauze pad moistened in the sterile water.

- Dry the skin with a sterile 4x4 gauze.

- Apply a clean trach dressing and change the tube holder/tie if needed.

- Throw away all of the disposable supplies.

- Wash your hands.

Tracheostomy Tube Change

Tracheostomy tubes are to be changed monthly, or as needed, to decrease the chance of infections. You should always have a back-up trach tube, one the same size and one a size smaller. **Do Not change the trach tube unless you have had proper training.** It is very important to use sterile technique during the trach change procedure.

Equipment Needed:

- Sterile tracheostomy tube

- Sterile gloves

- Sterile water soluble lubricant

- Sterile towel

- Suction equipment

- 10 cc syringe

- Ambu bag

- Sterile 4x4 gauze

- Trach tube holder

- Trach dressing

- Hydrogen Peroxide

Procedure:
- Wash hands using proper technique

- Open the sterile kit and use the sterile towel wrapper for sterile field.

- Place sterile content on sterile field.

- Put on the sterile glove on your dominant hand.

- New trach tube should be deflated fully. Do not touch anything with the new tube to contaminate it.

- Remove the inner cannula from the new trach and replace it with the obturator.

- Put 10cc of air into the cuff using syringe and check for holes.

- Use water soluble lubricant to lubricate the tip of the tube. **Do not use petroleum based product.**

- Suction the patient if he or she needs suctioning.

- If the patient has a cuffed trach, deflate fully.

- Remove the trach tie or holder and the dressing.

- Clean the skin with sterile gauze 4x4 and sterile water.

- Disconnect the client from off the ventilator. It may be necessary for someone else to vent the patient with the ambu bag while you change the trach.

- Remove the trach tube with a downward, forward motion.

- Use your sterile hand to insert the new tube, gently, within 15-20 seconds, keeping the obturator in place.

- **Immediately remove the obturator.**

- Place the inner cannula into the trach tube.

- Inflate the cuff with the use of the minimal leak technique or with a cuff manometer.

- Check for adequate air exchange by putting your hand over the cannula opening. If there is no exchange of air, remove the trach **immediately and use ambu bag to vent the patient**, it is not in the trachea.

- Stabilize the tube with one hand until it is well secured in place with a tie or holder.

- Reconnect the patient to the ventilator once the tube is properly in place and secured.

- Dress trach site.

- Dispose of all remaining supplies.

- Wash your hands after removing gloves.

Early Warning Signs
It is very important for you to know the signs and symptoms of problems/infection.

Signs of Infection and causes:

- Changes in the color of the sputum, odor, volume and consistency.

- Lack of proper hand-washing and the use of dirty equipment are the main cause of infections.

- Improper suctioning.

- Improper trach change.

- Improper care of the stoma.

Breathing Symptoms

- Increased shortness of breath.

- Coughing increased

- Wheezing increased

- Respiratory rate increased

- Accessory muscle use.

Signs of Infection and causes cont'd…

- Sputum color change to yellow, green, tan or brown.

- Quantity and consistency of sputum change.

- Sputum bloody.

Other Signs And Symptoms
- Fever

- Rapid weight loss

- Loss of appetite

- Sleepiness

- Hands and feet swollen

- Headache

- Dizziness

- Anxiety or confusion

- Visual problems

- Cyanosis

Call the physician for any changes/problems.
If problems or symptoms are severe, call **911**.

SUCTIONING

Coughing removes secretions from the airway. Some patients are unable to cough strongly enough to produce sputum, which prevents the lungs from getting the oxygen they need. Suctioning removes the secretions from the airway, allowing the patient to breathe better.

You may use sterile or clean technique to do suctioning. When a patient needs to be suctioned, he or she may begin to breathe noisily, or begin to cough, or if on a ventilator, the high pressure alarm will go off (Breath of Life 2009).

REMEMBER
- Always wash your hands before and after suctioning.
- Always wear gloves when suctioning.
- Follow sterile or clean technique.
- Follow Company protocol.
- Inform physician of any signs and symptoms of infection or any changes.

Nebulizer

What is a nebulizer treatment?

1. A nebulizer treatment ("Neb") gives medicine as a fine mist that is breathed into the lungs. This is done by using a specific machine ("nebulizer").

2. Nebs must be given as instructed in order for them to work.

Who needs an aerosol treatment?

People with respiratory problems, such as Asthma, COPD, Pneumonia, or other respiratory issues may need aerosol treatment. Small muscular tubes in the lungs called bronchioles help move air deep into the lungs, where oxygen is taken into the blood. In asthma there tubes get plugged or they tighten, making it very difficult to breathe.

Asthma medication opens up the airway to allow the person to breathe easier.

Asthma can be worsened by emotional stress, physical exercise chest colds, coughing, wheezing or going from a warm environment to a cold one.

How to set up nebulizer.

1. Explain what you are going to do before you do it.

2. Place the machine on a level surface. It may vibrate during use, so keep it away from the edge of the table.

3. Keep it off the floor for good air circulation and to keep the filter clean longer.

4. Plug the power cord into a 3-prong outlet.

Procedure <u>**FOLLOW PROCEDURE FOR MEDICATION PASS (6 rights of medication and proper hand washing)**</u>

1. Pour the solution into the cup.

2. Put the top on the neb cup and attach a face mask or mouthpiece.

3. Hold the neb cup in an upright position for the whole treatment.

4. Connect one end of the air tubing to the machine and the other to the bottom of the neb cup.

5. For the Mouthpiece – place it over the tongue and between the teeth. You should be able to see the mist at the opposite end disappear as the medicine is inhaled.

6. Continue until all of the medicine is gone from the neb cup (About 10 minutes).

7. You will hear a sputter and see a decrease in the amount of mist coming out.

8. When this happens, tap on the neb cup gently to get the rest of the medicine back to the bottom of the neb cup.

9. Always have an unopened neb kit as a backup

Care of a nebulizer:

1. All parts of the disposable nebulizer, except the tubing, are cleaned after each treatment. (see Diagram).

2. With power switch on "off" unplug power cord from the wall outlet.

3. Disconnect tubing from the air inlet connector and set aside.

4. Disassemble mouth piece or mask from cup. Open chamber by turning cap counter clockwise.

5. Wash all items except tubing under warm running water.

6. Air dries all pieces on a clean paper towel.

7. Do not towel dry nebulizer parts. This could cause contamination.

8. Never place any nebulizer part in an automatic dishwasher. Doing so could cause damage.

Note:

1. Entire used disposable nebulizer kit should be changed monthly.

2. The changing of the nebulizer kit should be documented.

3. The zip-lock bag should be labeled with the name of the resident and the date the new nebulizer package was opened.

4. **Always keep an extra nebulizer kit on hand at all times**

Filter Change:

1. Filter should be change every three month or sooner if filter turns gray in color.

2. Filter should be inspected every week.

3. Remove filter cup cap by grasping it firmly and pulling it out of the unit.

4. Remove dirty filter with fingers and discard.

5. Additional filters should always be kept on hand.

6. Push filter cap with new filter into position.

7. Reusing filter or substituting any other material such as cotton for a filter will result in compressor damage.

8. The date the filter was changed should be documented.

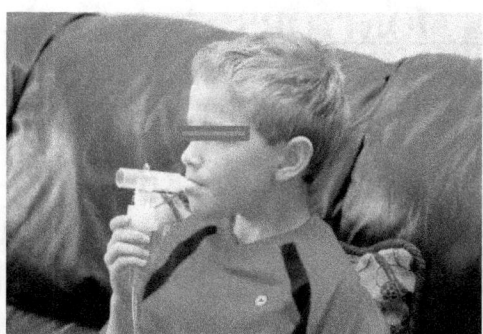
Nebulization by mouth

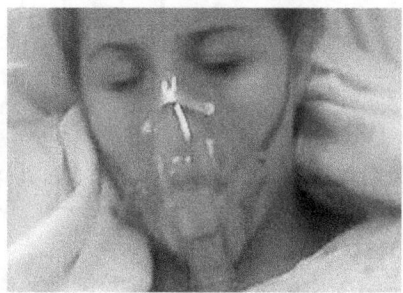
Nebulization by mask

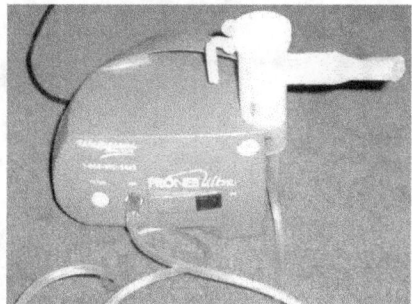
Nebulizer machine

INFANT APNEA MONITORS

Home Apnea Monitors are portable machines used to monitor a person's heart beat and breathing. Infants with breathing problems due to congenital disease are usually placed on home apnea monitors.

This machine monitors the baby's heartbeat and breathing. If breathing stops for 20 seconds, or if the heart rate gets down below acceptable levels, an alarm goes off, alerting the nurse to immediately provide airway intervention. The monitors have both audible and lighted alarms, and health care professionals need to be trained in infant CPR techniques.

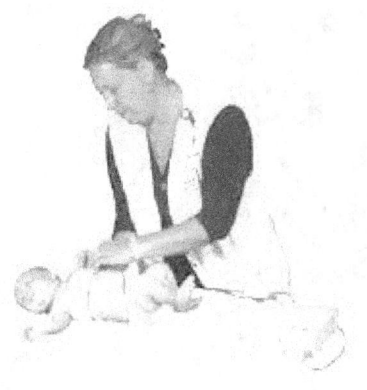

VENTILATORS

A ventilator is a machine that supports a client's breathing due to respiratory insufficiency or respiratory failure. Special tubing is connected to the vent and also connected to the client's tracheostomy. The tube carries air, which could be oxygenated, from the ventilator to the lungs.

A ventilator uses pressure to blow air or a mixture of oxygen and air into the lungs. This pressure is known as positive pressure. The ventilator can be programed to exchange air at set number of times a minute. Sometimes it is set so that the client can trigger the machine to deliver air into the lungs. If the client fails to trigger the ventilator within a certain amount of time, the machine automatically delivers air to keep the client breathing. This is SIMV mode of ventilation (synchronized intermittent mandatory ventilation). That means the machine will deliver breaths at the volume and rate set, and the client can take spontaneous breaths at a volume and rate controlled by them.

The machine won't attempt to deliver breaths until the client is done exhaling. Some people who are on ventilators are able to eat, drink, and talk.

Clients with the need to sustain life with the use of a ventilator require a competent nurse with current knowledge and experience of the latest medical technology. The nurse should also have the ability to work with patients and their families who are experiencing the challenges associated with life with a ventilator.

The home care nurse will receive training from a respiratory specialist from the company that supplies the ventilator. The specialist will set up the ventilator as prescribed by the pulmonologist, and will maintain the equipment on a regular basis. The home care nurse should make sure he or she receives a thorough working knowledge of the particular vent he or she will be working with. Ask questions, take notes, and have hands-on demonstrations. The suppliers of the ventilator want the home care nurse to be competent and confidence, therefore, they will ensure that the nurse is thoroughly trained.

Maintenance of the ventilator is available twenty-four hours per day, seven days per week. There is contact information readily available, and it is usually posted on the equipment itself.

There has to be a back-up ventilator for emergency. The nurse's duties include checking the equipment at the start of the shift, including checking the back-up ventilator to make sure it is working as it should, and that all settings remain as ordered and programed.

Since there are many different kinds of ventilators, it is practical to get trained on the kind of ventilator each client has. Below are two pictures of ventilators.

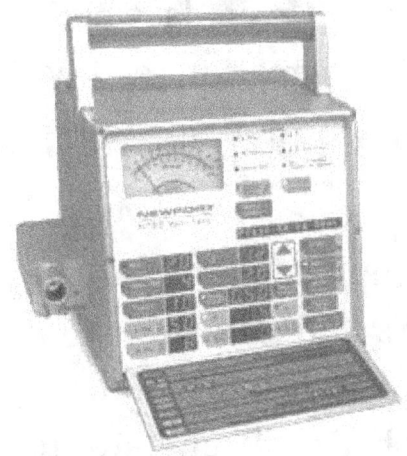

Newport HT50 Ventilator
(Notice the opening to the left where the tubing should be connected.)

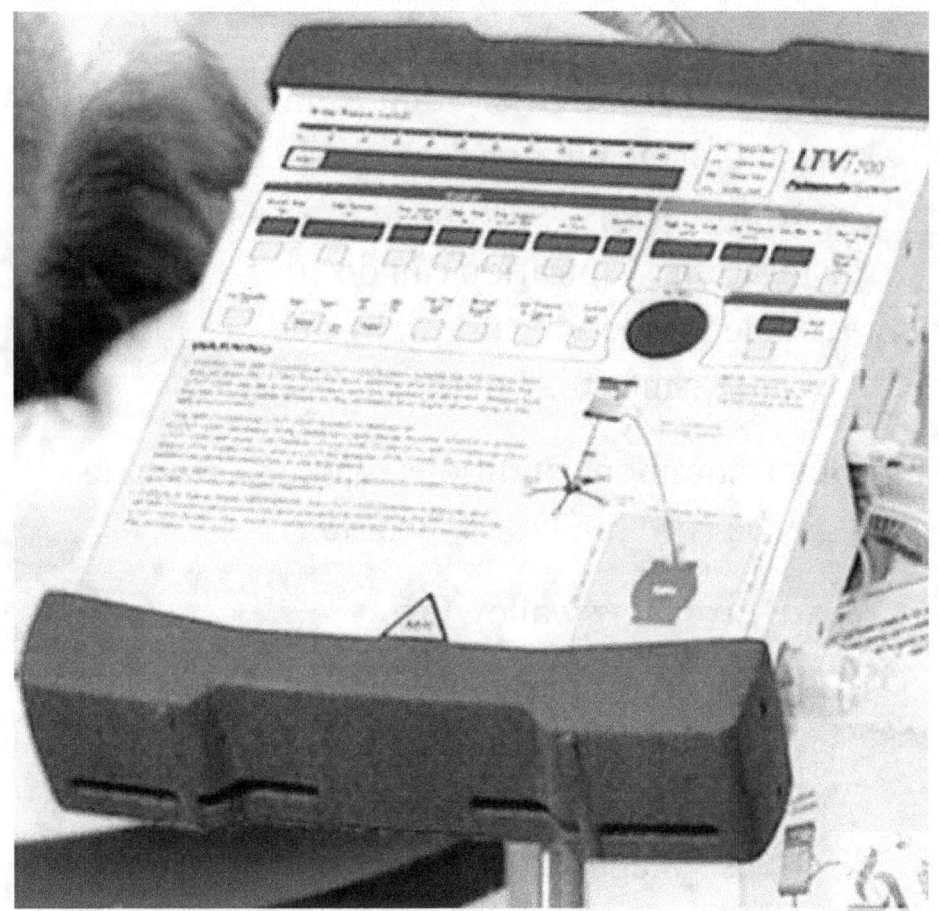

LTV-1200 Ventilator
(The tubing is connected to the right.)

GASTROSTOMY TUBES

A gastrostomy tube or g-tube may be a good choice for children or adults who are unable to eat and drink enough to meet their daily nutrition needs. A g-tube may also help prevent aspiration. Aspiration can occur if a person has trouble swallowing normally and breathe food or liquids into the lungs.

Some common conditions in which a g-tube may be recommended include:

- Problem swallowing
- Stroke
- Mouth or esophagus cancer
- Esophagus diseases
- Birth defects

A g-tube may be placed if there is a long-term condition that will not allow swallowing. In some cases, such as a minor stroke from which a person may recover, a g-tube may not be permanent (Yale Medical Group 2013).

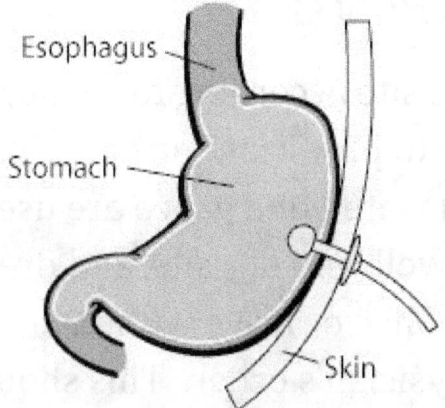

Gastrostomy Tube Placement

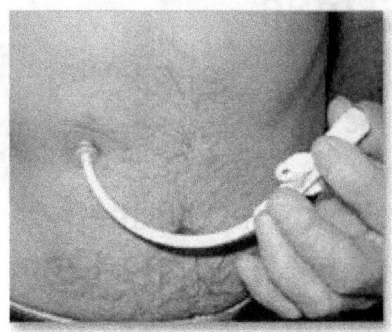

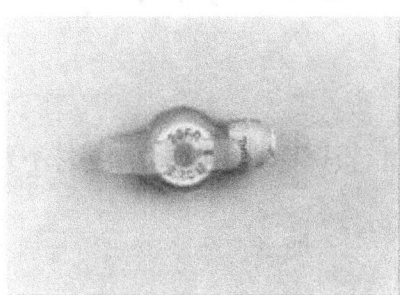

Mic-key Button G-tube (Pediatric)

CARE OF THE G-TUBE SITE

Clean client's g-tube site according to agency policy, or according to physician's order. Generally, soap and water, and gauze are used to clean site. Rinse well, and dry site, and dress with gauze drain sponge or leave without dressing; follow physician's order. This should be done at least twice per day or as necessary, or according to physician's order.

GASTROSTOMY TUBE FEEDING

Gravity Feeding Method (Rockcastle Regional Hospital 2009):

- Fill the feeding bag with the prescribed amount of formula and run the fluid to the end of the tube to clear out any air. Clamp the tube.

- Connect the end of the feeding bag tubing to the G-tube.

- Hang the bag at least 18 inches above the level of your G-tube.

- Open the clamp and allow the formula to flow into the G-tube.
- Follow with the prescribed amount of water.

- After each feeding, rinse the bag and tubing. Every 24 hours, wash with soapy water and rinse thoroughly.

Pump Feeding Method

Fill the feeding bag with the prescribed amount of formula and run the fluid to the end of the tube to clear out any air. Clamp the tube.

- Connect the end of the feeding bag tubing to the G-tube. Set the pump rate of flow to the prescribed rate per hour.

- Open the clamp on the tubing; press the start button on your pump.

- When feeding is complete, disconnect the feeding set.

- Connect the tip of an empty syringe to the feeding tube and slowly push in the prescribed amount of water.

After each feeding, rinse the bag and tubing. Every 24 hours, wash with soapy water and rinse thoroughly.

Syringe Feeding Method

- Remove the plunger from a syringe and connect the syringe to the G-tube.

- Hold the syringe upright and pour the formula into the syringe.

- Refill the syringe as the formula reaches the bottom of the syringe

- Repeat the process until the prescribed amount of formula is given.

- Follow the feeding with the prescribed amount of water.

After each feeding, rinse the bag and tubing. Every 24 hours, wash with soapy water and rinse thoroughly.

HOME IV INFUSION/ELASTOMETRIC DEVICES

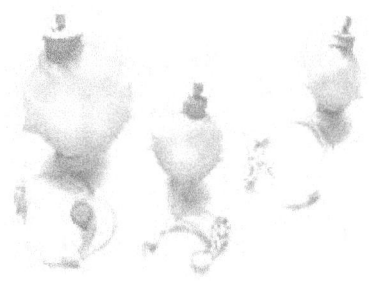

Elastomeric IV delivery systems - various sizes

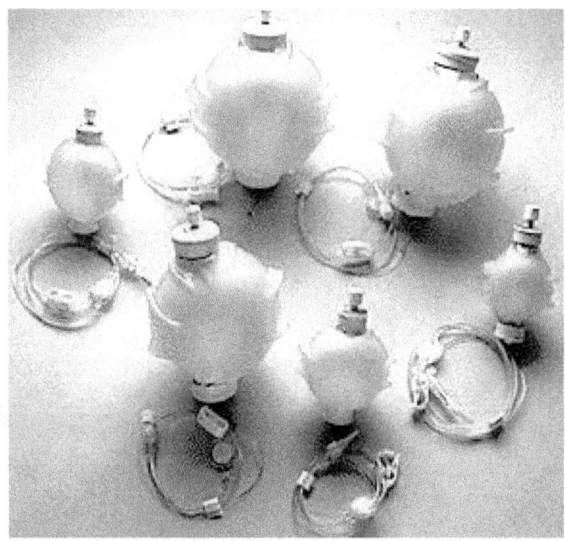

Elastomeric IV delivery systems – various sizes

Elastomeric infusion pumps

These are infusion devices that have disposable containers with inner elastic bladders, filled with medication.

Elastomeric (balloon) pressure administers medication, and capillary tubing or a glass orifice in the IV set regulates the flow.

The Elastomeric infusion system is indicated for antibiotic therapy.

Some also are indicated for continuous infusion of medication for chemotherapy and pain management through intravenous, inter-arterial, subcutaneous or epidural routes.

They are ideal for both ambulatory patients and patients receiving home or alternate site care, and are simple and safe to use for pharmacists, nurses and patients alike.

PART 6

SAFETY IN THE HOME

Safety of the patient is of the utmost importance. Whether in the hospital, in an institution, or in a person's home, safety is a top priority. Safety involves every aspect of patient care, including the client's environment.

Air quality and toxic substance are problems encountered in clients' homes in the USA every day. These elements should be addressed when the initial assessment is done, since they are associated with numerous negative health outcomes (Gershon RRM 2008).

There are several patient safety organizations in the USA. One such organization is the National Patient Safety Foundation (NPSF), a voice for patient safety since 1997 (T. N. Foundation 2012). This organization is made up of several individuals including patients, families, researches, providers , and the community (T. N. Foundation 2012).

"The National Patient Safety Foundation Research Grants Program seeks to stimulate new, innovative projects directed toward enhancing patient safety in the United States" (T. N. Foundation 2012).

Safety in the client's home includes the nurse doing thorough physical assessments. Detailed assessments may prevent the development of more serious medical problems.

Infection control should also be considered as safety precaution. Hand washing before and after caring for the client is essential in helping to prevent infection. Practicing and teaching good personal hygiene to the patient and family will also provide good outcome in infection control efforts.

The initial assessment of a client includes the client's mental status. Determination is made as to the need for a caregiver, if a client lives alone.

Assessment of the client's environment is also done. This means the agency nurse who sees the client for the first time has to fulfill certain safety criteria set forth by the State. These criteria may differ from State to State.

Areas that are covered include assessment of the bathroom for hand rails, safety bath mat, and shower chair or whether there is a need for any other accessories. The assessment of the environment should also include whether there is a fire extinguisher, fire sprinkler and alarm, and if they are functioning adequately. There are guidelines, as mentioned above, that the nursing agency provides as a part of the documentation that are completed by the nurse at the initial assessment.

Prevention of medication errors is another safety matter of the utmost importance. Preparing medication with distractions such as talking to others, listening to the radio, talking on the phone or doing anything that is distracting may cause medication errors.

Preparing medication in poor lighting may also cause medication errors.

Nurses and caregivers who are certified by their State to administer medication need to adhere to the above precautions. Additionally, the six rights of medication administration must be followed (the right client, right medication, right dose, right time, right route and right documentation).

Safety is not limited to what is mentioned in this handbook. Also, remember safety assessment is on-going. Follow agency policies and procedures as set forth by the State.

CLIENT ABUSE

The client in home care should be assessed for any signs of abuse. Unfortunately, abuse of a client may happen anywhere, including in his or her own home. The abuse may come from other members of the household, as well as caregivers.

According to an article by Geiger-Brown, et al, which was sited in "Home Health Care Patients and Safety Hazards in the Home", the writer did a thorough review of the risks and risk factors for violence in home care.

Studies have found that the most common reported form of abuse is verbal (Gershon RRM 2008). There are signs that may indicate abuse of the patient.

Verbal abuse is to belittle, reprimand or humiliate a person, causing emotional distress. Signs of verbal abuse include rocking, sucking or mumbling (Corporation n.d.).

This may be hard to prove, however, if there are suspicions one should contact Adult Proactive Services (APS) for further investigations. There laws in place to protect adults and disabled persons from abuse. Each county has an APS agency.

Physical abuse "means knowingly causing physical harm or recklessly causing serious physical harm to a patient by physical contact with the patient or by use of physical or chemical restraint, medication, or isolation as punishment, for staff convenience, excessively, as a substitute for treatment, or in amounts that preclude habitation and treatment." (T. C. Foundation 2002). Signs of physical abuse are:

- **"An injury that is not immediately reported to the patient's family**. A caretaker responsible for an injury is strongly tempted to hide the injury from the patient's family.

- **A burn of any kind**. Patients should never be burned or scalded. Caretakers should guarantee that a patient's environment is free of burn risk.

- **Multiple bruises of similar shape**. Repeated strikes with a belt, electrical cord or other objects usually cause similarly shaped bruises.

- **Non-reaction to pain**. Patients who are repeatedly subjected to physical abuse may eventually stop showing any outward reaction or response." (General n.d.)

Neglect of patients includes the following:

- "Weight loss and weight gain. Every substantial change in weight should have a medical explanation.

- Poor dental care. A lack of dental care can lead to other, more serious medical problems.

- Poor physical hygiene. Cleanliness is absolutely essential to good health… (General n.d.).

- Pressure sores that do not heal. Pressure sores are almost always avoidable and curable.

- Torn or dirty clothes. A facility that does not have adequate resources to properly care for patients may do the laundry less frequently.

- Unusual requests for food, such as begging for something to eat or asking for food immediately after a served meal. Busy caretakers may fail to notice that a patient has lost the ability to get food from a plate to his mouth." (General n.d.).

ABUSE AMONG HEALTH CARE WORKERS

Abuse among health care workers occurs sometimes. According to Jeanne Geiger-Brown, PhD, RN and company, there is a link between abuse by healthcare workers and depression.

Home care workers provide care without protection. A study describes the frequency of abuse and violence experienced by workers in home care and its relationship to workers' depression. Violence was highly associated with depression, according to one survey (Jeanne Geiger-Brown, PhD, RN n.d.). Preventive and early intervention measures should be implemented to reduce abuse and violence among home care workers due to mental health issues (Jeanne Geiger-Brown, PhD, RN n.d.).

DISASTER PLANNING IN HOME CARE

"The National Association for Home Care &Hospice (NAHC) Emergency Preparedness Workgroup was established to develop an all hazards emergency preparedness plan to be used by home care and hospice providers" (Hospice 2008).

"Federal, state and local governments have created universal emergency and disaster planning standards for health care organizations. Government units such as Homeland Security, the Federal Emergency Management Agency, and the Centers for Disease Control, in concert with State and County public health or health and human service units have developed these standards. Government expects health care organizations to adopt and implement a standard planning protocol so that in the event of a disaster or emergency resources are maximized to best respond to a specific incident" (Hospice 2008).

On admission, the admitting home care nurse will assign each patient a priority code, indicating the patient's emergency rating (Hospice 2008).

The admitting nurse will obtain contact phone numbers, and educate on emergency planning options with the patient and family.

All information will be placed in the patient's chart in paper format as well as electronic format (Hospice 2008).

At the time of admission, each patient will be given a list of items to have available for use in the event of an emergency.

Patients requiring power for life support equipment will be registered with local utility companies, and with local emergency agencies. The patients and family members will receive education to assist them in managing emergencies (Hospice 2008).

A list of vendors who supply patients' medical supplies will be obtained and kept in the patients' charts (Hospice 2008).

Bibliography

Breath of Life Home Health Equipment and Respiratory Services. *Breath of Life.* 2009. http://www.bolhme.com/education/TracheostomyCare&Suctioning.pdf.

Corporation, York Law. *York Law Corporation.* n.d. http://www.yorklawcorp.com/practice/nursing-home-abuse/verbal-abuse (accessed August 29, 2012).

Foundation, The Cleveland Clinic. *Abuse and Neglect of Patients and Misappropriation of Patient's Property for Subacute & Rehabilitation.* June 20, 2002. http://www.clevelandclinic.org/socialwork/abuse_and_neglect_of_patients_an.htm (accessed August 30, 2012).

Foundation, The National Patient Safety. *Patient Safety ListServ.* 2012. http://www.npsf.org/for-healthcare-professionals/resource-center/ (accessed August 27, 2012).

General, Office Of The Indiana Attorney. *What to do if you suspect patient abuse or neglect.* n.d. http://www.in.gov/attorneygeneral/2360.htm (accessed August 30, 2012).

Gershon RRM, Pogorzelska M, Qureshi KA, et al. *Home Health Care Patients and Safety Hazards in the Home.* 2008. http://www.ncbi.nlm.nih.gov/books/NBK43619/ (accessed August 29, 2012).

Hospice, The National Association for Home Care &. *EMERGENCY PREPAREDNESS PACKETFOR HOME HEALTH AGENCIES.* 2008. http://www.nahc.org/regulatory/ep_binder.pdf (accessed September 3, 2012).

Jeanne Geiger-Brown, PhD, RN. *Abuse and Violence During Home Care Work as Predictor of Worker Depression.* n.d. http://www.in.gov/attorneygeneral/2360.htm (accessed August 30, 2012).

K.Cervisio. *Home Healthcare Nurse.* 2010.

Mayo Clinic . *Mayo School of Health Science .* 2012. http://www.mayo.edu/mshs/careers/nursing.

National Association for Home Care & Hospice. *National Association for Home Care & Hospice 2013 Legislative Blueprint for Action.* 2012. http://www.congressweb.com/nahc/docfiles/NAHC%202013%20Legislative%20Blueprint%20for%20Action%20(2013%20Legislative%20Priorities)%20(Home%20Health%20Legislation%201980-2012).pdf (accessed May 5, 2013).

Online Education Database. *Home Health Care Nurse.* 2012. http://oedb.org/fast-track-careers-nursing/home-health-care-nurse.

Rockcastle Regional Hospital. *Rockcastle Regional Hospital Respiratory Care Center.* 2009. http://www.rockcastleregional.org/education/library/healthsheet.php?id=3,86493.

Swanson, B. "Careers in Health Care." 140-141. 2005.

Wikipedia. *Home Care.* May 2, 2012. http://en.wikipedia.org/wiki/Home_care.

Wyatt Matas & Associates. *How Home Healthcare Thrives with Healthcare Reform.* October 22, 2010. http://www.doctorsmakinghousecalls.com/wp-content/uploads/2011/09/Wyatt-Matas-White-Paper-How-Home-Healthcare-Thrives-with-Healthcare-Reform-Final.pdf (accessed May 5, 2013).

Yale Medical Group. *Yale School Of Medicine.* 2013. http://www.yalemedicalgroup.org/stw/Page.asp?PageID=STW035271 (accessed May 5/5/13, 2013).

APPENDIX

COPIES OF SOME DOCUMENTATION FOR HOME HEALTH CARE INITIAL ASSESSMENT ARE INCLUDED. FORMS MAY VARY DEPENDING ON THE AGENCY, AND STATE REQUIREMENTS:

PATIENT BILL OF RIGHTS & RESPONSIBILITIES

All patients with home health care services, or their families, possess basic rights and responsibilities. These include:

THE RIGHT TO:

1. Be treated with dignity, consideration and respect.
2. Have services/products and equipment available directly or by contract.
3. Be informed of organization ownership and control.
4. Have any specific charges for services to be paid by client and those charges covered by insurance, third-party payment or public benefit programs.
5. Be informed of billing policies, payment procedures and any changes in the information provided on admission as they occur within 30 days from the date that the organization is made aware of changes.
6. Receive care from professionally trained personnel. To know the names, discipline and responsibilities of the people giving you care and the frequency of visit or visits proposed to be furnished. To have the right of choice in care providers.
7. Receive information in a manner that you can understand and have access to interpreters as indicated and necessary to ensure accurate communication.
8. Right to participate in the plan of care and/or any change in the plan before the change is made.
9. Know the home care service's policy on client advance directives, before care is provided, including a description of the individual's right under State Law (whether statutory or as recognized by the courts of the State) and how such rights are implemented by the home care service.
10. Know how to make a complaint or recommended changes in home care service policies and services, and have the freedom to do so.
11. Receive service without regard to race, creed, gender, age, handicap, sexual orientation, veteran status or lifestyle.
12. Receive service without regard to whether or not any advance directive has been executed.
13. Participate in designing a care plan for your needs, and periodically updating it as your condition changes.
14. Be notifies in advance of treatment options, transfers, when and why within a reasonable time frame of anticipated termination of service.
15. Receive and access services consistently and in a timely manner in accordance with organization's stated operational policy.
16. Education instructions and requirements for continuing care when the services of the agency are discontinued.
17. Participate in the selection of options for alternative levels of care or referral to other organizations, as indicated by the client's need for continuing care.
18. Be referred to another provider organization if the organization is unable to meet the client's needs or if the client is not satisfied with the care they are receiving.
19. Be able to voice grievances regarding treatment, care or respect for property that is or fails to be furnished by anyone services on behalf of the organizations without reprisal for doing so.

**Averel Carby
Home Health Care, LLC**

**ADMISSION CONSENT/
SERVICE AGREEMENT**

PATIENT NAME:_____ MR#_____ DATE_____
ADDRESS:_____

PATIENT RIGHTS & RESPONSIBILITIES

I hereby certify that I have been given a copy of The Patient Bill of Rights and Responsibilities, and a copy of notice of Privacy, and a copy of Privacy Act Statement (The Privacy Act of 1974).

CONSENT FOR TREATMENT

I hereby consent for Averel Carby, RN, to administer treatment as is ordered while under my Physician's Plan of Treatment. I hereby certify I fully understand the need for my consent for such treatment, as explained to me and I also certify that no guarantee or assurance has been made to me as to the results that may be obtained. I also understand that I have the right to assist the Home Care Service in planning of my care while under this Home Care Service. I understand that if I do not fulfill my responsibilities the Home Care Service may notify me and terminate my care.

RELEASE OF INFORMATION

I understand that Averel Carby, RN, may use or disclose protected health information about me to carry out treatment, payment or health care operations. Averel Carby, RN may release information to or receive information from insurance companies, health plans, Medicare, Medicaid or any other person or entity that may be responsible for paying or processing for payment any portion of my bill for services; any person or entity affiliated with or representing for purposes of administration, billing, and quality and risk management; any hospital, nursing home, or other health care facility to which I may be/have been admitted; any assisted living or personal care facility of which I am a resident; any physician providing my care; family members and other caregivers who are part of my plan of care; licensing and accrediting bodies (i.e. JCAHO, CHAP), and other health care providers in order to initiate treatment.

I would be willing to have a surveyor visit in my home with advance telephone notice by the Agency:☐Yes ☐No

ADVANCE DIRECTIVES

I have received the information on Advance Directives, including the information on my right as a resident to accept or refuse medical or surgical treatment. This includes information on Patient Self Determination Act; written description of the State Law; and written description of my rights under the Patient Self Determination Act of 1990. I have received this facility's written policies respecting the implementation of my rights under the Patient Self Determination Act of 1990 and State Law: (Mark all the apply.)

I have executed an Advance Directive? ☐Yes ☐No (if yes, provide a copy to the Home Care Service)

☐ Individual Instruction/Living Will
☐ Power of Attorney for Health Care/Healthcare Surrogate

**Averel Carby
Home Health Care, LLC**

ADMISSION CONSENT/ SERVICE AGREEMENT

AUTHORIZATION FOR PAYMENT

I consent to the release of all records required to act on this request. I consent for any holder of medical or other information about me to release that said information to the Social Security Administration, or its intermediary or carriers, Medicaid and/or my private insurance company, in order to process any claim(s) or related claim(s), or as set forth in the Notice of Privacy Practices or in accordance with the Health Insurance Portability and Accountability Act of 1996. I certify that the information given by me in applying for payment under Title XVIII of the Social Security Act is correct. I request that payment of authorized benefits and medical information be made to the above named Home Health Care Service.

Service	Freq. Plan	Medicare ☐	Medicaid ☐	Insurance Specify	Charge
Skilled Nursing		100%	100%		
Home Health Aide		100%	100%		
Physical Therapy		100%	100%		
Occupational Therapy		100%	100%		
Speech Therapy		100%	100%		
Medical Social Services		100%	100%		
Other:					
Medical Supplies Specify:					

Based on communication with your insurance carrier, your policy covers _____ % on home health benefits. You will be responsible for any deductible and the remaining % of the bill.

Total Visits Per Week: _____
Total Charges Per Week: _____
Out of Pocket Expense Per Week: _____

CONSENT TO PHOTOGRAPH

I hereby give my consent to the agency and its agents and employees to take pictures for medical documentation purposes. They may be released to the Social Security Administration, or its intermediaries or carriers, Medicaid and/or my private insurance company, in support of my request for payment.

> I understand a copy of this consent form shall be as valid as the original and shall remain in effect until I am discharged from the agency. I also understand that I may revoke this consent in writing at any time.

Consent must be signed by the patient or nearest relative or legal guardian in the case of a minor or when the patient physically unable or mentally incompetent to sign the form.

_____   _____
Patient's Signature   Responsible Person or Legal Guardian Signature

_____   _____
Witness Signature/Home Care Service Representative   Printed Name & Relationship of Person above

☐ Patient unable to sign due to: _____

On-the-go Vitals™ presents Book: "The Nurse's Guide to Home Health Care"
©All Rights Reserved
http://www.allhealthacademy.com

BRADEN SCALE FOR PREDICTING PRESSURE SORE RISK IN HOME CARE

NPO[1]: Nothing by mouth | IV[2]: Intravenously | TPN[3]: Total parenteral nutrition

					DATE OF ASSESSMENT 1	2	3	4
SENSORY PERCEPTION Ability to respond meaningfully to pressure-related discomfort	**1. Completely Limited:** a. Unresponsive (does not moan, flinch, or grasp) to painful stimuli, due to diminished level of consciousness or sedation. **OR** b. Limited ability to feel pain over most of body.	**2. Very Limited:** a. Responds only to painful stimuli. Cannot communicate discomfort except by moaning or restlessness **OR** b. Has a sensory impairment which limits the ability to feel pain or discomfort over 1/2 of body.	**3. Slightly Limited:** a. Responds to verbal commands, but cannot always communicate discomfort or the need to be turned. **OR** b. Has some sensory impairment which limits ability to feel pain or discomfort in 1 or 2 extremities.	**4. No Impairment:** Responds to verbal commands. Has no sensory deficit which would limit ability to feel or voice pain or discomfort.				
MOISTURE Degree to which skin is exposed to moisture	**1. Constantly Moist:** Skin is kept moist almost constantly by perspiration, urine, etc. Dampness is detected every time patient is moved or turned.	**2. Often Moist:** Skin is often, but not always moist. Linen must be changed as often as 3 times in 24 hours.	**3. Occasionally Moist:** Skin is occasionally moist, requiring an extra linen change approximately once a day.	**4. Rarely Moist:** Skin is usually dry; linen only requires changing at routine intervals.				
ACTIVITY Degree of physical activity	**1. Bedfast:** Confined to bed.	**2. Chairfast:** Ability to walk severely limited or non-existent. Cannot bear own weight and/or must be assisted into chair or wheelchair.	**3. Walks Occasionally:** Walks occasionally during day, but for very short distances, with or without assistance. Spends majority of day in bed or chair	**4. Walks Frequently:** Walks outside bedroom twice a day and inside room at least once every 2 hours during waking hours				
MOBILITY Ability to change and control body position	**1. Completely Immobile:** Does not make even slight changes in body or extremity position without assistance	**2. Very Limited:** Makes occasional slight changes in body or extremity position but unable to make frequent or significant changes independently.	**3. Slightly Limited:** Makes frequent though slight changes in body or extremity position independently.	**4. No Limitation:** Makes major and frequent changes in position without assistance.				
NUTRITION Usual food intake pattern	**1. Very Poor:** a. Never eats a complete meal. Rarely eats more than 1/3 of any food offered. Eats 2 servings or less of protein (meat or dairy products) per day. Takes fluids poorly. Does not take a liquid dietary supplement **OR** b. Is NPO[1] and/or maintained on clear liquids or IV's[2] for more than 5 days.	**2. Probably Inadequate:** a. Rarely eats a complete meal and generally eats only about 1/2 of any food offered. Protein intake includes only 3 servings of meat or dairy products per day. Occasionally will take a dietary supplement. **OR** b. Receives less than optimum amount of liquid diet or tube feeding.	**3. Adequate:** a. Eats over half of most meals. Eats a total of 4 servings of protein (meat, dairy products) per day. Occasionally will refuse a meal, but will usually take a supplement when offered **OR** b. Is on a tube feeding or TPN[3] regimen which probably meets most of nutritional needs.	**4. Excellent:** Eats most of every meal. Never refuses a meal. Usually eats a total of 4 or more servings of meat and dairy products. Occasionally eats between meals. Does not require supplementation.				
FRICTION AND SHEAR	**1. Problem:** Requires moderate to maximum assistance in moving. Complete lifting without sliding against sheets is impossible. Frequently slides down in bed or chair, requiring frequent repositioning with maximum assistance. Spasticity, contractures or agitation leads to almost constant friction	**2. Potential Problem:** Moves feebly or requires minimum assistance. During a move skin probably slides to some extent against sheets, chair, restraints or other devices. Maintains relatively good position in chair or bed most of the time but occasionally slides down.	**3. No Apparent Problem:** Moves in bed and in chair independently and has sufficient muscle strength to lift up completely during move. Maintains good position in bed or chair.					
				TOTAL SCORE				
					Initials	Initials	Initials	Initials

1 Signature

2 Signature

3 Signature

4 Signature

SCORE KEY:
15-18 = Mild Risk
13-14 = Moderate Risk
10-12 = High Risk
≤ 9 = Severe Risk

Patient/Resident Name

ID# (if applicable)

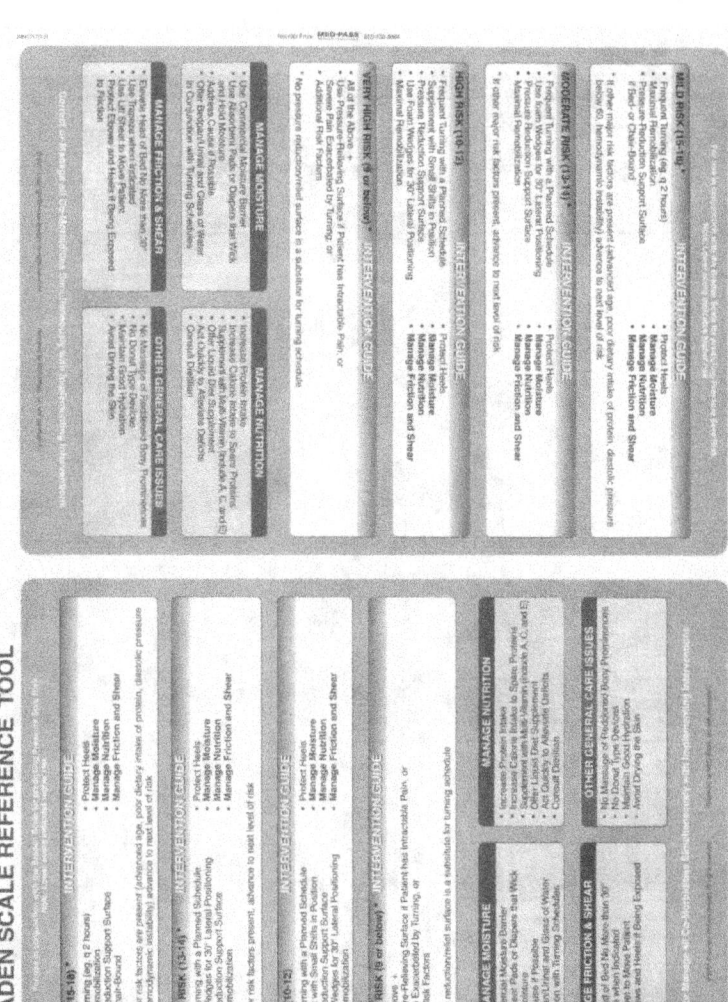

SKILLED NURSING INITIAL EVALUATION/ASSESSMENT

RED Ink = Specific 485 items (completed per agency policy)

Date	Time In	Time Out

Patient Name (First, MI, Last) | ID No. | **2** SOC Date | **3** Certification Period From / To

24 Primary Physician's Name | Address | Physician's Phone

THE FOLLOWING ARE TO BE DISCUSSED WITH THE PATIENT AND/OR CAREGIVER PRIOR TO PROVISION OF CARE

- ☐ Rights/Responsibilities
- ☐ Charges for Services/Assign Of Benefits
- ☐ Complaint Procedure & Hotline Number
- ☐ Services Provided/Anticipated Freq./Duration of Visits
- ☐ Fire/Safety/Disaster & Emergency Plan
- ☐ Advance Directive
- ☐ Pt./Caregiver Development of Care Plan
- ☐ Goals of Visits
- ☐ Discharge Planning
- ☐ Privacy Notice

DIAGNOSIS

17 ALLERGIES: ☐ NKA ☐ Allergic to: _____ Birth Date: _____

11 Primary Diagnosis | ICD-9-CM | Comments
Date: ___ O/E

Other Pertinent Diagnoses | ICD-9-CM
a. Date: O/E
b. Date: O/E
c. Date: O/E
d. Date: O/E

12 Surgical Diagnosis | ICD-9-CM
a. Date:
b. Date:

20 PROGNOSIS: ☐ Poor ☐ Fair ☐ Good | **21** Is the patient DNR "Do Not Resuscitate"? ☐ Yes ☐ No | Comments

21 Terminal Care Intervention: Assess/Perform/Instruct Pt/Cg   A   P   I   Additional Orders (Specify)
- ☐ Spiritual, grieving & coping methods
- ☐ S/S of impending death
- ☐ Notification procedures for death at home
Comments

Advance Directives: ☐ Yes ☐ No | Comments
Intent: ☐ DNR ☐ Medical Power of Attorney ☐ Living Will ☐ Other
Copies on File at Agency? ☐ Yes ☐ No   Copy requested? ☐ Yes ☐ No   Result:

Patient/Family Knowledge and Coping Level Regarding Present Diagnosis: Patient: _____ Family: _____

High Risk Factors | Comments
- ☐ Alcohol dependency ☐ Obesity ☐ Chronic conditions
- ☐ Heavy smoking ☐ Drug dependency ☐ Cultural/Religious practices that may impact care

LIVING ARRANGEMENTS

Emergency Contact Person: Name: _____ Phone: _____
(Outside of the house)

Household Composition: | Comments
☐ Lives Alone ☐ With Spouse or Significant Other ☐ Other Family Member ☐ With Friend ☐ Other
Marital Status: ☐ Single ☐ Married ☐ Widowed ☐ Divorced ☐ Separated ☐ Unknown
Family Supportive: ☐ Yes ☐ No

Caregiver Name: _____ Relationship: _____

Caregiver able/willing to provide all care ☐ Yes ☐ No | Comments
Caregiver able to receive/follow instructions ☐ Yes ☐ No
Caregiver able/willing to assist with ADLs and needed care ☐ Yes ☐ No

18A FUNCTIONAL LIMITATIONS:
- ☐ Amputation ☐ Paralysis ☐ Legally Blind
- ☐ Bowel/Bladder Incontinence ☐ Endurance ☐ Dyspnea with minimal exertion
- ☐ Contracture ☐ Ambulation ☐ Other (specify):
- ☐ Hearing ☐ Speech

Homebound ☐ No ☐ Yes: Reason:
- ☐ Need assistance for all activities
- ☐ Residual weakness
- ☐ Requires max. assistance/taxing effort to leave home
- ☐ Confusion, unsafe to go out of home alone
- ☐ Unable to safely leave home unassisted
- ☐ Severe SOB, SOB upon exertion
- ☐ Other (specify)

Additional Orders (Specify): _____ Comments

Safety/Sanitation Hazards affecting patient: (Mark all that apply.) | Comments
- ☐ Stairs ☐ Inadequate lighting, heating and cooling ☐ Insects/rodents infestation
- ☐ Narrow or obstructed walkways ☐ Lack of fire safety devices ☐ Cluttered/soiled living area
- ☐ No gas/electric appliance ☐ No running water, plumbing ☐ Other (specify):

Patient Name (First, MI, Last) | ID No.

1 of 6

LIVING ARRANGEMENTS (continued)

15 SAFETY MEASURES:
- ☐ Anticoagulant Precautions
- ☐ O₂ Precautions
- ☐ Slow Position Change
- ☐ Proper Position During Meals
- ☐ Use of Assistive Devices
- ☐ Support During Transfer and Ambulation
- ☐ Emergency Plan Developed
- ☐ Demonstrates knowledge and understanding of safety measures/safety management ☐ Yes ☐ No
- ☐ Equipment Use/Safety
- ☐ Keep Side Rails Up
- ☐ Keep Pathways Clear
- ☐ Safety in ADLs
- ☐ Seizure Precautions
- ☐ Standard Precautions/Infection Control
- ☐ Neutropenic Precautions
- ☐ Fall Precautions
- ☐ Other _____

Triage/Risk Code (Agency specific) _____
Disaster Code (Agency specific) _____
Comments _____

FINANCIAL: Ability of Patient to handle Personal Finances:
☐ Independent ☐ Needs Assistance ☐ Totally Dependent
- ☐ Medical expenses not covered by Insurance/Medicare
- ☐ Inadequate to buy necessities (Food, Medications, Supplies, etc.)
- ☐ Inappropriate use of limited income (Buying non-essentials - Alcohol, Junk food, etc.)

Comments _____

Community Agencies/Social Service Screening	Yes	No	Comments
Community Resource Info needed to manage care			
Altered affect (i.e. depression, grief, body image chg.)			
Suicide Ideation			
Suspected Abuse/Neglect, I.e.: (Please circle) unexplained bruises, inadequate food, fearful of family member, Cg. exploitation of funds, sexual abuse, neglect, left unattended if needs constant supervision.			
Inadequate method to cook or shop for groceries			
MSW referral needed For?			
Coordinator notified			

SENSORY STATUS

VITAL SIGNS: PULSE: ☐ Apical _____ (Reg) (Irreg) Height _____ B/P Lying _____ Sitting _____ Standing _____
☐ Radial _____ (Reg) (Irreg) Weight _____   L
TEMP _____ RESP _____ ☐ Actual ☐ Stated   R

21 Notify Physician of Temperature Ranges > _____ or < _____
Known Recent Lab Results: _____

VISION: ☐ WNL ☐ Blurred Vision ☐ Contacts: R L ☐ Other _____ Comments _____
☐ Glasses ☐ Glaucoma ☐ Cataracts

EARS / NOSE / THROAT / MOUTH ☐ WNL
Hearing Loss? ☐ L ☐ R Aid Used? ☐ L ☐ R
Ear Pain? ☐ L ☐ R
Other: _____

Nasal Condition:
- ☐ WNL
- ☐ Congestion/Sinus Prob.
- ☐ Loss of smell
- ☐ Other

Pharyngeal Condition:
- ☐ WNL
- ☐ Hoarseness
- ☐ Sore throat
- ☐ Other

Mouth Condition: ☐ WNL
- ☐ Abnormal Oral Mucosa Appearance
- ☐ Gum problems ☐ Chewing problems
- ☐ Dentures ☐ Difficulty swallowing
- ☐ Other

21 EENT Interventions: Assess/Perform/Instruct Pt/Cg: A P I
- ☐ Methods to control Disequilibrium problems
- ☐ Instillation of Ear medications
- ☐ Instillation of Ophthalmic medications

Additional Orders (Specify) _____
Comments _____

COMMUNICATION ☐ WNL   YES NO
- Limited educational background ☐ Pt ☐ Cg
- Reading or writing problems ☐ Pt ☐ Cg
- Slow learner ☐ Pt ☐ Cg
- Speech/language barrier ☐ Pt ☐ Cg
- Primary language _____
- Interpreter needed?
- Motivated to learn? ☐ Pt ☐ Cg

Patient Learning Preferences:
☐ Literal ☐ Visual ☐ Demonstrative ☐ Graphic
☐ Verbal Instructions ☐ Other _____
Comments _____

Neurological ☐ WNL ☐ Dizziness ☐ PERRL
☐ Headache (Describe Location, Duration) _____
☐ Other _____
Comments: _____

21 Neurological Interventions: Assess/Perform/Instruct Pt/Cg: A P I
- ☐ Changes in LOC/Neurological Status
- ☐ Communication Skills
- ☐ Seizure Precautions
- ☐ Orientation Techniques: _____

Additional Orders (Specify) _____

MUSCULOSKELETAL ☐ WNL
- ☐ Limited ROM (give location) _____
- ☐ Bone or Joint problems _____
- ☐ Pain or Cramps _____
- ☐ Redness, Warmth, Swelling _____
- ☐ Decreased Mobility/Endurance _____
- ☐ Tremors _____
- ☐ Amputation of _____
- ☐ Prosthesis/Appliance _____

21 Musculoskeletal Interventions: Assess/Perform/Instruct Pt/Cg: A P I
- ☐ Positioning body alignment techniques & ROM exercises
- ☐ Cast Care
- ☐ Circulatory checks as applicable
- ☐ Adherence to appropriate activity levels

Additional Orders (Specify) _____
Comments _____

Patient Name (First, MI, Last) _____ ID No. _____

© 2003 MED-PASS, INC.   Reorder From: MED-PASS 800-438-8884   Form # HC1634H

SENSORY STATUS (continued)

Frequency of Pain interfering with patient's activity or movement:

☐ Patient has no pain or pain does not interfere with activity or movement ☐ Less often than daily ☐ Daily, but not constantly ☐ All of the time

PAIN PROFILE Primary Site ______

Intensity: 0 1 (LOW) 2 3 4 5 6 7 8 9 10 (HIGH)

Pain Description: ☐ sharp ☐ dull ☐ other ______

Onset Date: ______
Pain precipitated by: ______
Pain relieved by: ______
History of pain management: ______
Current pain management & effectiveness: ______
Patient's pain goal: ______
Progress toward pain goal: ______
Pain site assessment: ______

21 Pain Management Interventions: Assess/Perform/Instruct Pt/Cg: A P I

☐ ______ ☐ ☐ ☐
☐ ______ ☐ ☐ ☐
☐ ______ ☐ ☐ ☐

■ **See Pain Assessment/Documentation (per agency policy)**
Refer to: ______
Comments

INTEGUMENTARY STATUS

Skin Turgor: ☐ Good ☐ Fair ☐ Poor
Skin Color: ☐ Pink/WNL ☐ Pale ☐ Jaundice ☐ Cyanotic
Skin: ☐ Dry ☐ Diaphoretic ☐ Warm ☐ Cool
Skin: ☐ Wounds ☐ Ulcers ☐ Incision ☐ Rashes
☐ Ostomy ☐ Other

Comments

Nails: ☐ Normal ☐ Problems

Instructed on Standard Precautions: ☐ Yes ☐ No

Instructed on measures to control infections: ☐ Yes ☐ No

INTEGUMENTARY STATUS LOCATOR Key: 1 - Skin Lesion 2 - Pressure Ulcer 3 - Stasis Ulcer 4 - Surgical Wound

Type	Location	Size	Drainage	Amount	Odor	Stage	Surrounding Skin

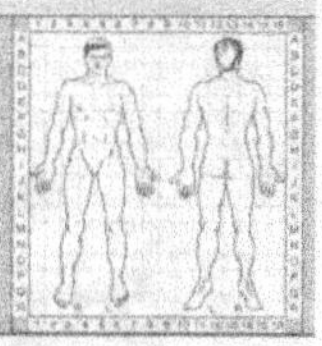

21 Integumentary Interventions: Assess/Perform/Instruct Pt/Cg: A P I

☐ Wound care as follows: ______ ☐ ☐ ☐

☐ Stoma care: ______ ☐ ☐ ☐

☐ Incisional care: ______ ☐ ☐ ☐

☐ S/S of complications, infection to include: ______ ☐ ☐ ☐

☐ Other: ______ ☐ ☐ ☐

RESPIRATORY STATUS

RESPIRATORY ☐ WNL ☐ Cough ______ ☐ Smoker ______ ☐ Sputum ______ ☐ Orthopnea ______

☐ Breath Sounds ______ ☐ Hemoptysis ______ ☐ Cyanosis ______ ☐ Tracheostomy (size) ______

☐ Other ______ Comments

21 Respiratory Interventions: Assess/Perform/Instruct Pt/Cg: A P I

☐ Respiratory Status ☐
☐ Methods to recognize Pulmonary Dysfunction & relieve complications ☐ ☐ ☐
☐ O_2 Administration at ______ L/Min; Via ______ ☐ ☐ ☐
Care of O_2 Equipment: Safety Precautions
☐ Notify Physician of Respiratory Ranges > ______ or < ______

☐ Post Operative Respiratory Precautions (T/C/DB) ☐ ☐ ☐
☐ Nebulizer Inhalation Treatment with ______ ☐ ☐ ☐
☐ Suctioning Technique ☐ ☐ ☐
☐ Trach Care ☐ ☐ ☐
☐ Chest Physiotherapy ☐ ☐ ☐
☐ Pulse Oximetry per Symptomology ☐ ☐ ☐

Additional Orders (Specify): ______

CARDIOVASCULAR STATUS

Cardiovascular: ☐ WNL **12** ☐ Pacemaker ___/___/___ (Date inserted)

☐ Palpitations ☐ Fatigues easily ☐ Poor Capillary Refill
☐ Chest pain ☐ Other: (specify) ______

Heart Rate: ☐ WNL
☐ Regular ☐ Irregular ☐ Reg./Irreg.
☐ Tachycardia ☐ Braycardia

☐ **Edema:** ☐ Pedal R/L ☐ Dependent ______
☐ Pitting +1 /+2 /+3 /+4 (site) ______
☐ Non-pitting (site) ______

Comments

21 Cardiovascular/Hematological Interventions: Assess/Perform/Instruct Pt/Cg A P I

☐ Cardiovascular Status ☐
☐ Measures to recognize Cardiac Dysfunction and relieve complication ☐ ☐ ☐
☐ Notify Physician of Systolic > ______ and < ______ ☐ ☐
Diastolic > ______ and < ______
☐ Notify Physician of Pulse Rate > ______ and < ______ ☐ ☐

☐ Weigh patient q ______ ☐ ☐ ☐
☐ Notify Physician of weight variation of ______ lbs. ☐ ☐
☐ Methods to detect/alleviate Fluid Retention ☐ ☐ ☐
☐ Methods to recognize Vascular Dysfunction & relieve complications ☐ ☐ ☐
☐ Methods to detect/alleviate Hematological Disorders ☐ ☐ ☐

Additional Orders (Specify): ______

Patient Name (First, MI, Last) | **ID No.** | 3 of 6

© 2005 MED-PASS, INC. Reorder From: MED-PASS 800-438-8884 Form # HC1034H

RENAL/GENITOURINARY STATUS

URINARY ☐ WNL Urinary Color _____ Amt _____ Odor _____ Comments _____
☐ Hematuria ☐ Oliguria ☐ Polyuria ☐ Burning
☐ Retention ☐ Cramping/Dysuria/Sediment ☐ Incontinence

REPRODUCTIVE/GENITAL
☐ Problems with Lumps/Breast Discharge ☐ Lack of Monthly Breast Self Examination
☐ Problems with Menses/Menopause ☐ Discharge from Vagina/Penis
☐ Abnormal Pap Smear ☐ Prostate Problems

External Genitalia:
☐ Normal ☐ Abnormal
Per: ☐ Physical Assessment ☐ Pt/Cg reported
Comments _____

☐ Pregnant: EDC _____

Renal/Genitourinary Interventions: Assess/Perform/Instruct Pt/Cg: A P I
☐ Fluid Intake at _____ ml per day   ☐☐☐
☐ Bladder Training to include _____   ☐☐☐
☐ Catheter Care   ☐☐☐
☐ Ileal Conduit Care to include _____   ☐☐☐
☐ Foley Irrigation   ☐☐☐

☐ Catheter change q _____ with _____ F _____ ml balloon catheter   A P I
☐ Injections _____   ☐☐☐
  ☐ Nurse to administer/instruct pt/cg to administer
  _____ (Drug) _____ (Dose) _____ (Route)
  _____ (Drug) _____ (Dose) _____ (Route)
  _____ (Drug) _____ (Dose) _____ (Route)

Additional Orders (Specify): _____

ENDOCRINE ☐ WNL   Comments _____
☐ Polyuria/Polydipsia/Polyphagia ☐ Thyroid Disease Able to draw up insulin ☐Y ☐N
☐ Neuropathy/Radiculopathy ☐ Diabetes Able to administer insulin ☐Y ☐N
☐ Urine Testing Performed ☐ Insulin Dependent? How Long? _____
☐ Blood Sugar Glucometer Use Most recent FBS _____
☐ Oral Hypoglycemic Agent
☐ Additional Information/Needs _____

Endocrine Interventions: Assess/Perform/Instruct Pt/Cg: A P I
☐ Use of electronic Glucose measuring device   ☐☐☐
☐ Diabetic care to include diet, activity, stress, foot care, skin care   ☐☐☐
☐ S/S of complications of Diabetes   ☐☐☐
☐ S/S of Hypo/Hyperglycemia   ☐☐☐
☐ Preparation/administration of Insulin   ☐☐☐

☐ Prefill Syringes q _____ per Physician Order   A P I
☐ Monitor glucometer recordings for variations & compliance   ☐☐☐
☐ Notify Physician of blood sugar over _____ and under _____ MG%   ☐☐☐
☐ Glucometer testing to be performed by _____ q _____

Additional Orders (Specify): _____

GASTROINTESTINAL STATUS

☐ Nausea/Vomiting ☐ Abdominal Distention or Tenderness Comments _____
☐ Abdominal Pain ☐ Enteral Feedings
☐ Abnormal Stool Characteristics Type/Tube _____ Size _____
☐ Diarrhea/Constipation Changed _____ Formula _____
☐ Use/Abuse of Laxatives Amt _____ Freq _____
☐ Stool Incontinence ☐ Flow Control Device
☐ Absent or Minimal Bowel Sounds ☐ Ostomy Location _____
☐ Abdominal Masses ☐ Problems Associated with Ostomy

Bowel: ☐ WNL Last BM _____ Usual Frequency _____   ☐ Diarrhea ☐ Abnormal stools: Gray/Tarry/Fresh blood
☐ Constipation: Chronic/Acute/Occasional ☐ Lax/enema use: Type _____   ☐ Hemorrhoids: Internal / External

Digestive/Gastrointestinal Interventions: Assess/Perform/Instruct Pt/Cg: A P I
☐ _____ diet compliance   ☐☐☐
☐ Measuring/Recording intake and output   ☐☐☐
☐ Methods to promote Oral Intake   ☐☐☐
☐ Measures to recognize dysfunction and relieve complications   ☐☐☐
☐ Parenteral Nutrition and the care/use of equipment to include _____   ☐☐☐
☐ Enteral Nutrition and the care/use of equipment to include _____   ☐☐☐
☐ Gastrostomy Tube (specify) _____   ☐☐☐

☐ NG Tube (specify) _____   A P I
☐ Bowel Training Program   ☐☐☐
☐ Ostomy Care to include _____   ☐☐☐
☐ Change feeding tube _____ using size _____ q _____   ☐☐
☐ Digital Exam/relieve fecal impaction; give Fleet's/SS enema as needed   ☐☐

Additional Orders (Specify): _____

NUTRITION/HYDRATION   ☐ Diet _____   Comments _____
☐ Impaired/Inadequate Fluid Intake ☐ Dentures? ☐ Upper ☐ Lower   ☐ Gross Obesity
☐ Impaired/Inadequate Food Intake ☐ Recent Weight Gain or Loss – Amt _____   ☐ Received Enteral/Parenteral Nutrition
☐ Difficulty Chewing/Swallowing (Reason) _____   ☐ Impaired Healing of Complex Wound
☐ Compliant with Ordered Diet ☐ Yes ☐ No   ☐ Nutritional Risk ☐ High
☐ Lactating/Breast Feeding   ☐ Mod ☐ Low

NUTRITIONAL REQUIREMENTS NEW OR CHANGED:
☐ _____ Sodium Diet ☐ Calorie ADA Diet ☐ Bland Diet ☐ Mechanical (Soft, Hi-Fiber, etc.) ☐ NG Tube
☐ _____ Protein Hi Diet ☐ _____ / Low Diet ☐ Regular ☐ PEG Tube
☐ _____ Carbohydrate Hi Diet ☐ _____ / Low Diet ☐ Supplement ☐ _____ Tube
☐ Enteral Feeding ☐ Other (Specify) _____
Amount _____ ml/day Pump Type _____

Patient Name (First, MI, Last) _____   ID No _____

NEURO/EMOTIONAL/BEHAVIORAL STATUS

PSYCHOLOGICAL STATUS/BEHAVIOR ☐ WNL ☐ Anxiety ☐ Agitation ☐ Depression
☐ Difficulty Coping w/Altered Health Status ☐ Other ____________

Comments

19 MENTAL STATUS:
☐ Oriented ☐ Comatose ☐ Forgetful ☐ Agitated
☐ Depressed ☐ Disoriented ☐ Lethargic
☐ Other ____________

21 Psychiatric Nursing Intervention: Assess/Perform/Instruct Pt/Cg

	A	P	I
☐ Suicide Precautions	☐	☐	☐
☐ Counseling	☐	☐	☐
☐ Grief Management	☐	☐	☐

Additional Orders (Specify): ____________

ADLs/IADLs

	INDEP	ASSIST Some	ASSIST Max		INDEP	ASSIST Some	ASSIST Max	Comments
Personal Care: tub, shower, sponge	☐	☐	☐	Medication: ability to take	☐	☐	☐	
Toileting: bowel/bladder	☐	☐	☐	Shopping	☐	☐	☐	
Ambulation	☐	☐	☐	Light Housekeeping	☐	☐	☐	
Transfers	☐	☐	☐	Laundry	☐	☐	☐	
Stairs	☐	☐	☐	Using Phone	☐	☐	☐	
Dressing: Upper, lower	☐	☐	☐	Handling Money	☐	☐	☐	
Eating	☐	☐	☐	Other: ______	☐	☐	☐	
Full meal preparation	☐	☐	☐					
Light snack preparation	☐	☐	☐	Home Health Aide Needed	☐ Yes	☐ No		

18B ACTIVITIES PERMITTED: ☐ Complete bed rest ☐ Up as tolerated ☐ Exercise prescribed ☐ Independent at home ☐ Cane ☐ Walker
☐ Bed rest with BRP ☐ Transfer bed-chair ☐ Partial weight bearing ☐ Crutches ☐ Wheelchair ☐ Other ____________

MEDICATIONS

10 MEDICATIONS: DOSE/FREQUENCY/ROUTE ☐ See Medication Profile **Note:** See Med Profile Addendum for Drug Regimen Review per Agency Policy

☐ **IV Access Present** ☐ Peripheal ☐ PICC ☐ Central: Define ____________ Date Inserted: ____________

Comments

21 High Tech/Special Procedures: Assess/Perform/Instruct Pt/Cg

	A	P	I
☐ Administration of ________ IV medication) in ________ (solution) to run at ______ ml/hr via ________ (Pump / Gravity)	☐	☐	☐
☐ Flush IV/PICC/Midline with 5-10ml of NS before and after antibiotic infusion. Follow with 3-5ml Heparin ____U/ml flush	☐	☐	☐
☐ Change ________ dressing q ________ and PRN using sterile techniques with alcohol/betadine	☐	☐	☐
☐ Change injection cap q ________ and PRN	☐	☐	☐
☐ Flush ________ catheter with ________	☐	☐	☐
☐ Change Huber needle q ______ and PRN using sterile technique	☐	☐	☐
☐ Access port q ______ and PRN to flush with ________	☐	☐	☐
☐ Pump/Equipment (specify) ________	☐	☐	☐
☐ Equipment use/Safety	☐	☐	☐
☐ Start Peripheal IV and maintain site, q ______ or q ______ days and PRN for s/s of infiltration/infection	☐	☐	☐
☐ S/S of infiltration and emergency procedures	☐	☐	☐
☐ Other: ________	☐	☐	☐

Additional Orders (Specify): ____________

EQUIPMENT

	Present	Needs	N/A		Present	Needs	N/A		Present	Needs	N/A
☐ Hospital Bed	☐	☐	☐	☐ Transfer Equipment	☐	☐	☐	☐ Catheter	☐	☐	☐
☐ Trapeze	☐	☐	☐	☐ Bathroom Safety Devices	☐	☐	☐	☐ Pacemaker	☐	☐	☐
☐ Wheelchair	☐	☐	☐	☐ Grab Bars	☐	☐	☐	☐ Hearing Aid	☐	☐	☐
☐ Pressure Relieving Device	☐	☐	☐	☐ Tub Stool	☐	☐	☐	☐ Dentures	☐	☐	☐
☐ Suction Machine	☐	☐	☐	☐ Bedside Commode	☐	☐	☐	☐ Glasses/Lenses	☐	☐	☐
☐ Infusion Pump	☐	☐	☐	☐ Toileting Aids	☐	☐	☐	☐ Prosthetic Device	☐	☐	☐
☐ Oxygen	☐	☐	☐	☐ Hospital Bed	☐	☐	☐	☐ Leg Brace	☐	☐	☐
☐ Ambulation Aids	☐	☐	☐	☐ Dressing Aids	☐	☐	☐	☐ Ramps/Railings	☐	☐	☐
☐ Walker	☐	☐	☐	☐ Colostomy/Ileostomy Bags	☐	☐	☐	☐ Other	☐	☐	☐
☐ Cane	☐	☐	☐	Comments							
☐ Crutches	☐	☐	☐								

14 DME AND SUPPLIES:

DME:
☐ Bedside Commode ☐ Hospital Bed ☐ Walker
☐ Cane ☐ Tub/Shower Bench ☐ Other ____________
☐ Elevated Toilet Seat ☐ Wheelchair
☐ Grab Bars

DISPOSABLES:
☐ Diabetic Supplies ☐ Catheter Supplies
☐ Dressing Supplies ☐ Other (Specify) ____________
☐ IV Supplies

Comments

Patient Name (First, MI, Last) | ID No.

5 of 6

 Form # HC1034H

21 ORDERS FOR DISCIPLINE AND TREATMENTS

- ☐ SN visit frequency _____
- ☐ Assess VS & all body systems, knowledge of disease process and its associated care and treatment, med regimen knowledge, and S/S complications necessitating medical attention. _____
- ☐ Venipuncture for: _____
- ☐ May draw Labs from IV Access
- ☐ OTHER _____
- ☐ Implement and Instruct Standard Precautions/Infection Control
- ☐ Implement and Instruct Medication Regimen, including dosage, side effects, name, route, frequency, desired action & adverse reactions. _____
- ☐ Assess Medication Compliance/Med Set-up _____
- ☐ Management of disease process to include: _____
- ☐ HHA Visit Frequency _____ to assist w/personal care/ADLs/light housekeeping as needed
- ☐ PCA/R - Personal Care Aide/Respite Waiver Passport (circle one)
- ☐ PT to consult, evaluate and treat ☐ Physical Therapy Visit Frequency _____
- ☐ OT to consult, evaluate and treat ☐ Occupational Therapy Visit Frequency _____
- ☐ ST to consult, evaluate and treat ☐ Speech Therapy Visit Frequency _____
- ☐ MSW to evaluate and assess for needs ☐ Medical Social Worker Visit Frequency _____
- ☐ Supervision as follows: _____
- ☑ ☐ Dietitian evaluation.
- ☐ May accept orders from: Dr. _____ Dr. _____ Dr. _____

22 GOALS/REHABILITATION POTENTIAL/DISCHARGE PLANS

- ☐ The patient's safety will be enhanced throughout the home care service as evidenced by _____ within _____ period of time.
- ☐ The patient/caregiver will verbalize understanding of (disease process) _____ and all aspects of associated care within _____ period of time.
- ☐ The patient/caregiver will verbalize understanding of medications as evidenced by recall of action dose & side effects within _____ period of time.
- ☐ The patient/caregiver will verbalize understanding of _____ diet as evidenced by compliance with diet plan within _____ period of time.
- ☐ The patient's skin and mucous membranes will remain intact for this cert period.
- ☐ The patient's weight will be maintained between _____ and _____ for this cert period.
- ☐ The patient's _____ lab value will be within normal limits per physician assessment and patient's compliance with meds/diet this cert period.
- ☐ The patient's pain will be controlled and managed at the patient's own comfort level as verbalized by the patient/caregiver within _____ period of time.
- ☐ The patient's _____ catheter/ _____ tube will remain patent for this cert period.
- ☐ The patient's _____ infection will resolve as evidenced by _____ within _____ period of time.
- ☐ The patient's _____ site will be decreased in size to _____ cm or _____ % this cert period.
- ☐ The patient's home environment will be clean & safe, as evidenced by _____ within _____ period of time.
- ☐ The patient's hygiene and personal care needs will be met this cert period with the assistance of the home health aide.
- ☐ The patient will reach maximum functional potential, as evidenced by _____ within _____ period of time.
- ☐ The patient will have psycho/social needs met, as evidenced by _____ within _____ period of time.
- ☐ Rehabilitation potential _____
- ☐ Endpoint of daily visits

Discharge Plans ☐ Patient to be discharged when skilled care no longer needed ☐ Other (specify) _____
☐ Patient to be discharged to the care of: ☐ Self ☐ Caregiver ☐ Other: _____

Patient Strengths: ☐ Motivated Learner ☐ Strong Support System ☐ Absence of Multiple Disease Diagnosis ☐ Enhanced Socioeconomic Status ☐ Other _____
Conclusions: ☐ Skilled Intervention Needed ☐ Skilled Instruction Needed ☐ No Skilled Service Needed ☐ Other _____

PATIENT / CAREGIVER'S EXPECTATIONS: _____
Conference with: ☐ Other Staff Member _____ ☐ Physician Office _____ Re: _____

NURSING DIAGNOSIS: | **SKILLED SERVICES PROVIDED THIS VISIT AND PATIENT RESPONSE:**

23 60 Day Summary (Recertification Only)

Patient Signature (optional per HHA policy & procedures) _____ Patient Name _____ Record No. _____

25 Nursing Signature/Discipline and Date of verbal SOC where applicable: _____

On-the-go Vitals™ presents Book: "The Nurse's Guide to Home Health Care"
©All Rights Reserved
http://www.allhealthacademy.com

ASSESSMENTS (continued)

GI ☐ WNL
- ☐ Anomalies
- ☐ Absent Bowel Sounds
- ☐ N/V
- ☐ Diarrhea
- ☐ GE Reflux
- ☐ Emesis
- ☐ Constipation
- ☐ Bloody Stools
- ☐ Ostomy
- ☐ Distention
- ☐ Abdominal Tenderness
- ☐ Other _____

Patient wears diapers? ☐ Yes ☐ No
Patient is toilet trained? ☐ Yes ☐ No
☐ Stool: Color _____ Amount _____ Frequency _____

☐ Skilled Interventions: Assess/Perform/Instruct Pt/Cg: A P I
- ☐ diet compliance
- ☐ Measuring/recording intake and output
- ☐ Methods to promote oral intake
- ☐ Measures to recognize dysfunction and relieve complications
- ☐ Parenteral nutrition and the care/use of equipment to include:
- ☐ Enteral nutrition and the care/use of equipment to include:
- ☐ Gastrostomy tube (specify)
- ☐ NG tube (specify)
- ☐ Bowel training program
- ☐ Ostomy care to include
- ☐ Change feeding tube
  sizing size _____ tube q _____
- ☐ Digital Exam/relieve fecal impaction; give Fleets/SS enema

Additional Orders (Specify): _____

Comments: _____

GU/REPRODUCTIVE ☐ WNL
- ☐ Anomalies
- ☐ Renal/Bladder Diseases
- ☐ Polyuria
- ☐ Labial Lesions
- ☐ Circumcision
- ☐ Hypospadias
- ☐ Undescended Testes (before 3 yrs of age)
- ☐ Hydrocele
- ☐ Hematuria
- ☐ Vaginal Discharge
- ☐ Inguinal Hernia
- ☐ Hernia
- ☐ Other _____

URINE: Color _____ Amount _____ Frequency _____

☐ Skilled Interventions: Assess/Perform/Instruct Pt/Cg: A P I
- ☐ Fluid Intake at _____ ml per day
- ☐ Bladder training to include:
- ☐ Catheter care
- ☐ Ileal conduit care to include:
- ☐ Foley irrigation
- ☐ Catheter change q _____ with _____ F _____ ml balloon catheter
- ☐ Injections:
  - ☐ Nurse to administer/instruct pt/cg to administer

(time) (dose) (site)
(time) (dose) (site)

Additional Orders (Specify): _____

Comments: _____

NUTRITION
Diet/Formula: _____
Amount _____ Frequency _____
Route: ☐ Oral ☐ Bottle ☐ NG/GT/JT ☐ IV
       ☐ Breast

APPETITE: ☐ Good ☐ Anorexic
          ☐ Fair ☐ Food Allergies
          ☐ Poor

☐ Feeding observed during visit
Comments: _____

MUSCULOSKELETAL ☐ WNL
- ☐ Sydney Palm Crease
- ☐ Simian Crease
- ☐ Knock Knee/Pidgeon Toe
- ☐ Epiphyseal Enlargement
- ☐ Kyphosis
- ☐ Scoliosis
- ☐ Trendelenburg Gait
- ☐ Anomalies
- ☐ Fractures
- ☐ Cast/Splints
- ☐ Muscle Conditions/Diseases
- ☐ Poor Muscle Tone
- ☐ Contractures
- ☐ Limited Rom
- ☐ Poor Gross Motor Skills
- ☐ Poor Fine Motor Skills
- ☐ Other _____

☐ Skilled Interventions: Assess/Perform/Instruct Pt/Cg: A P I
- ☐ Positioning body alignment techniques & ROM exercises
- ☐ Cast care
- ☐ Circulatory checks as applicable
- ☐ Adherence to appropriate activity levels

Additional Orders (Specify): _____

Comments: _____

ENDOCRINE ☐ WNL
- ☐ Polyuria
- ☐ Polyphagia
- ☐ Abnormal Growth Pattern
- ☐ Abnormal Hair Texture/Distribution
- ☐ Abnormal Sexual Development
- ☐ Other _____

☐ Diabetic Insulin Dependent? ☐ Yes ☐ No

☐ Skilled Interventions: Assess/Perform/Instruct Pt/Cg: A P I
- ☐ Use of electronic Glucose measuring device
- ☐ Diabetic care to include: diet, activity, stress, foot care, skin care
- ☐ S/S of complications of Diabetes
- ☐ S/S of Hypo/Hyperglycemia
- ☐ Preparation/administration of Insulin
- ☐ Prefill Syringes q _____ per Physician Order
- ☐ Monitor glucometer recordings for variations & compliance
- ☐ Notify Physician of blood sugar over _____ and under _____ MG%
- ☐ Glucometer testing to be performed by _____ q _____

Additional Orders (Specify): _____

Comments: _____

Patient Name (First, MI, Last): _____ Record #: _____

ASSESSMENTS *(continued)*

CARDIOVASCULAR
☐ WNL

☐ Congenital Anomalies
☐ Cyanosis
☐ Pallor
☐ Murmur
☐ Petechiae
☐ Edema (Site ________)
☐ Poor Capillary Refill
☐ Umbilical Cord Abnormalities
☐ Hypertensive
☐ Other ________

Pulses: Pedal Pulses Present? ☐ Yes ☐ No

Skilled Interventions: Assess/Perform/Instruct Pt/Cg:	A	P	I
☐ Cardiovascular Status	☐	☐	☐
☐ Measures to recognize Cardiac Dysfunction and relieve complication	☐	☐	☐
☐ Notify Physician of Systolic > ______ and < ______ Diastolic > ______ and < ______	☐	☐	☐
☐ Notify Physician of Pulse Rate > ______ and < ______	☐	☐	☐
☐ Weigh patient q ______	☐	☐	☐
☐ Notify Physician of weight variation of ______ lbs.	☐	☐	☐
☐ Methods to detect/alleviate Fluid Retention	☐	☐	☐
☐ Methods to recognize Vascular Dysfunction & relieve complications	☐	☐	☐
☐ Methods to detect/alleviate Hematological Disorders	☐	☐	☐

Additional Orders (Specify): ________

Comments: ________

INFUSION
☐ Intermittent ☐ Continuous

Pump type: ________
Line type: ☐ Peripheral ☐ PIC ☐ Central
Line length: ______ cm Brand ________
Location: ________ Size: ________
# of Lumens: ________ Date inserted: ________
Date dressing last changed: ________
Site assessment: ☐ Clear ☐ Patent ☐ Drainage ☐ Redness ☐ Swelling

High Tech/Special Procedures: Assess/Perform/Instruct Pt/Cg:	A	P	I
☐ Administer IV fluids ______ at rate of ______ via ______ **Pump / Gravity** (circle one)	☐	☐	☐
☐ Change HL q 72 hours and PRN for infiltration/infection	☐	☐	☐
☐ Flush HL with ______ ml of normal Saline q ______	☐	☐	☐
☐ Flush HL with ______ ml of ______ unit/ml Heparin flush q ______	☐	☐	☐
☐ Use SASH (saline Antibiotic Saline Heparin) protocol	☐	☐	☐
☐ S/S of infiltration and emergency procedures	☐	☐	☐
☐ Change ______ catheter dressing ______ x a week using sterile techniques with alcohol/betadine	☐	☐	☐
☐ Change injection cap q ______ and PRN	☐	☐	☐
☐ Flush ______ catheter with ______	☐	☐	☐
☐ Change Huber needle 1 x a week and PRN using sterile technique	☐	☐	☐
☐ Access port 1 x a month and PRN to flush with ______	☐	☐	☐
☐ Port dressing change q ______ and PRN using sterile technique	☐	☐	☐
☐ PICC Line (Specify) ______	☐	☐	☐
☐ On ______ pump/equipment (Specify) ______	☐	☐	☐

Additional Orders (Specify): ________

Comments: ________

NEUROVASCULAR
☐ WNL

☐ Headaches
☐ Dizziness
☐ Spasms
☐ Abnormal Fontanels
☐ Seizures (describe) ________
☐ Tremors
☐ Neurological Disease
☐ Tetany
☐ Weakness
☐ Listlessness
☐ Irritability
☐ Fixed Pupils/Unequal Pupils
☐ Other ________

Patient's LOC ________
Reflexes appropriate for age? ☐ Yes ☐ No
Mental Behavioral Status: ________
Speech or Language Difficulties: ________
Cognitive Performance: ________
Social Skills: ________
Gross Motor Skills: ________
Fine Motor Skills: ________

Skilled Interventions: Assess/Perform/Instruct Pt/Cg:	A	P	I
☐ Changes in LOC/Neurological Status	☐	☐	☐
☐ Communication Skills	☐	☐	☐
☐ Seizure Precautions	☐	☐	☐
☐ Orientation Techniques:	☐	☐	☐

Additional Orders (Specify): ________

Comments: ________

RESPIRATORY
☐ WNL

☐ Rales
☐ Cough
☐ Retractions
☐ Crepitation
☐ Wheezing
☐ Clubbing
☐ Flaring
☐ Rhonchi
☐ Stridor
☐ Cyanosis ________
☐ Other ________

Skilled Interventions: Assess/Perform/Instruct Pt/Cg:	A	P	I
☐ Respiratory Status	☐	☐	☐
☐ Methods to recognize pulmonary dysfunction & relieve complications	☐	☐	☐
☐ O_2 Administration at ______ L/Min: Via ______ Care of O_2 Equipment: Safety Precautions	☐	☐	☐
☐ Notify Physician of Respiratory Ranges > ______ or < ______	☐	☐	☐
☐ Maintain Vent settings as Follows ______	☐	☐	☐
☐ Post Operative Respiratory Precautions (T/C/DB)	☐	☐	☐
☐ Nebulizer inhalation treatment with ______	☐	☐	☐
☐ Suctioning technique	☐	☐	☐
☐ Trach care	☐	☐	☐
☐ Chest physiotherapy	☐	☐	☐
☐ Pulse Oximetry per Symptomology	☐	☐	☐

Additional Orders (Specify): ________

Comments: ________

PAIN
Presence of Pain? ☐ Yes ☐ No
Pain Medication ________ Effective? ☐ Yes ☐ No

Pain Management Interventions: Assess/Perform/Instruct Pt/Cg	A	P	I
☐ ______	☐	☐	☐
☐ ______	☐	☐	☐
☐ ______	☐	☐	☐

WONG-BAKER FACES PAIN RATING SCALE
Use for non-communicative patients (patient should point to scale).

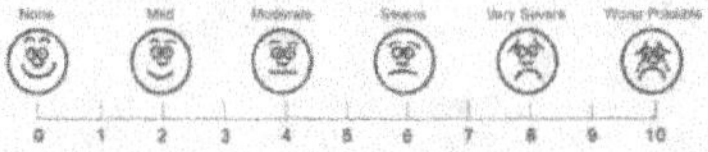

Additional Orders (Specify): ________

Comments: ________

Patient Name (First, MI, Last) ________ Record # ________

Form# HC1025H To order forms call: MED-PASS 800-438-8884 Page 4 of 6

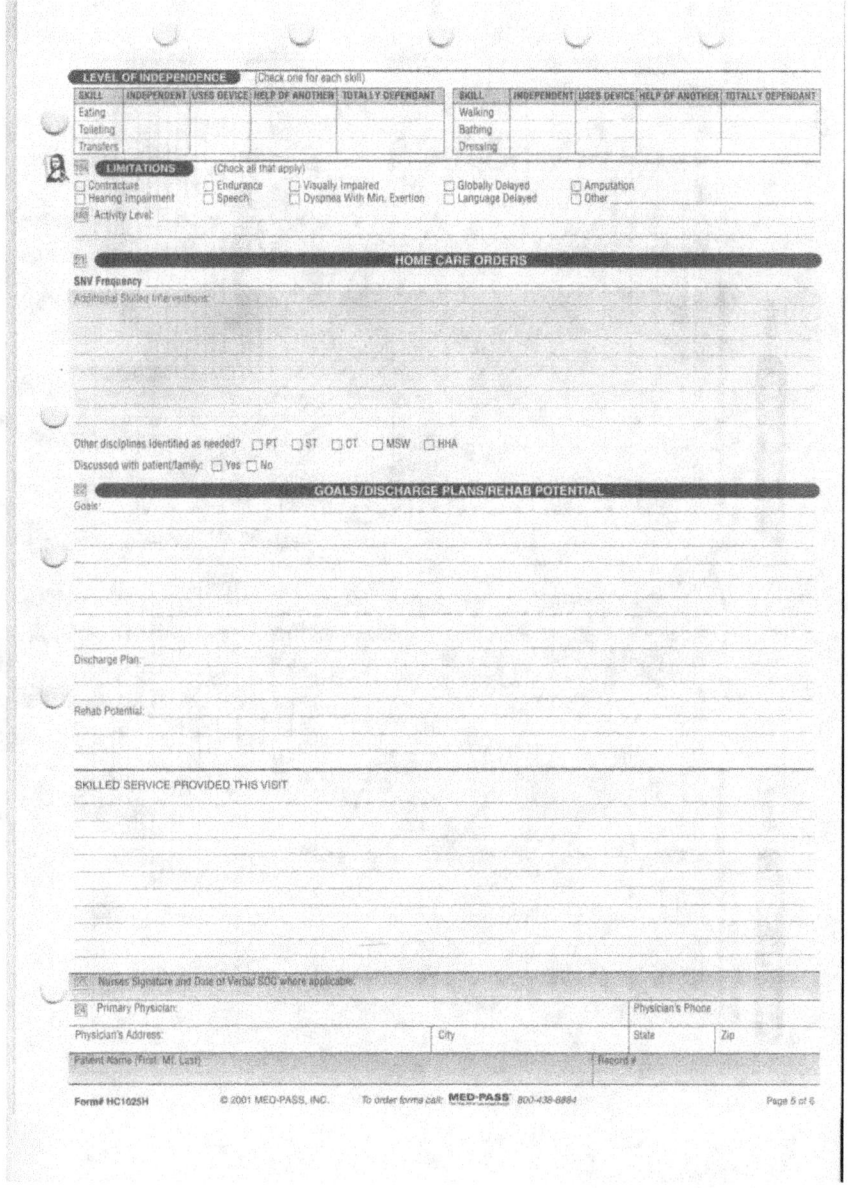

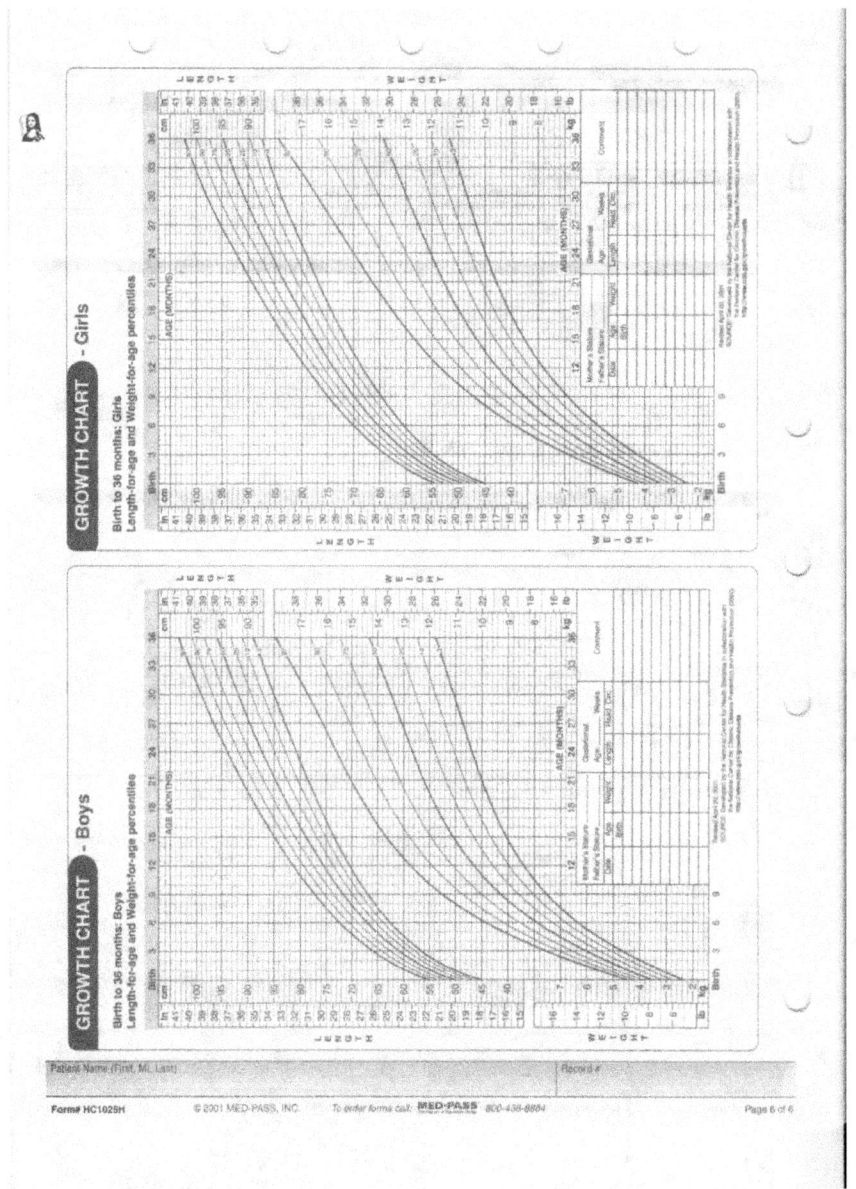

NOTES

NOTES

NOTES

NOTES

NOTES

NOTES

www.ingramcontent.com/pod-product-compliance
Lightning Source LLC
Chambersburg PA
CBHW081551170526
45166CB00009B/2656

9781491293034